THE 5-DAY MIRACLE DIET COMPANION

BY ADELE PUHN

The 5-Day Miracle Diet

*The 5-Day Miracle Diet
Companion*

THE 5-DAY MIRACLE DIET COMPANION

ADELE PUHN, M.S., C.N.S.

BALLANTINE BOOKS • NEW YORK

To Arthur
Whose love and wisdom balance my life;
and
In memory of my father,
the other man in my heart,
who showed me the poetry in life.

ACKNOWLEDGMENTS

My work doesn't just happen by itself. It grows instead like a sapling gently planted, watered, and nurtured. The soil most enriching for me is that which has always been tended by my husband, Arthur. I want once again to thank him for his unwavering support during the writing of *The 5-Day Miracle Diet* and the *Companion* book, and for the sixteen years we have been together. I appreciate his endless hours spent typing, reading, and editing. Arthur, my good friend, I love you.

I continue to be touched by the multitude of people who have opened their hearts and minds to the message of the 5-Day Miracle Diet. Thank you for taking the time to tell me what it has meant to you. It is your response that continues to fuel me in my commitment to freeing people from the tyranny of food.

To my clients, I apologize for my absence and thank you for your patience during the time I took to deliver my message to the world outside the office. I have appreciated your good-natured enthusiasm, input, and support. Experiencing your pain, joy, stories, dreams, and successes made it necessary to offer help to others who were not able to see me.

My love, thanks, and appreciation go to my dear children: Bonnee, David, Alyson, and Margot; and their respective spouses: Danny, Melissa, and Paul, for their ongoing encouragement and support. My only regret during this productive and busy time has been the limits placed on my ability to spend more time with them and my beautiful grandchildren: Charlotte, Lindsay, and Jake. I also have missed my mother-in-law, Sydelle Prince, who remains, as always, cheerful, supportive, and helpful in whatever circumstances arise. Thank you. The love for my family continues to nourish my heart, enabling me to continue the quest.

I appreciate and thank my agent, Wendy Weil, for her sage advice, encouragement, and her sense of humor throughout. Once again I thank Karla Doughtery for her remarkable ability in capturing my thoughts and translating my voice to the written page.

I have also been fortunate to be able to draw on the talents and enthusiastic support of the wonderful staff at Ballantine Books. I am grateful to Clare Ferraro for her continued interest and support. A large thank-you to my editor, Susan Randol, whose able mind polished this manuscript in record time as we rushed to press. I am greatly appreciative to the art department for the wonderful cover. I am extremely happy to be able to thank Jennifer Richards, my publicist at Ballantine, for her remarkable enthusiasm, hard work, and expertise. She continually amazes me with her energy, commitment, and dedication to the 5-Day Miracle Diet. To the rest of the Ballantine staff I give thanks for being the wonderful, supportive team that you are.

WELCOME TO MY WORLD

I'd like to share a secret with you: I never, ever thought that I would be a "thin" person. Throughout my childhood, the drama that enfolded around food, around cakes, doughnuts, and cookies, controlled my life. Never in my wildest dreams did I think that I could overcome the desire to eat these fattening, sugary foods. Worse, the doughnuts and the cookies kept me in a state of low blood sugar. I felt depressed, hopeless; I could never imagine leaving that apartment where food reigned supreme.

Even when I was a teenager and later a graduate student, food, if not the center of my life, was always prominent. I'd go on outrageous diets and lose weight—for four months. Then I'd gain it all back. I was the quintessential yo-yo: gaining, losing, and gaining again.

Basically, what I am sharing with you is the fact that I never imagined myself thin—as a child, as a student, and as a young adult! Never. It was so impossible a feat that it couldn't be a part of my dreams, even when I was sleeping.

Still there was always a piece of me, a serious, wish-with-all-my-heart place where I was thin. It was a place where I was more than thin: I was proud. There was a confidence to my demeanor. I felt I could do anything I wanted in the world, if I only put my mind to it.

Over time, that determination has helped this dare-not-say-aloud piece of me to become a reality. I'm slim, and I have so much energy and confidence that sometimes my husband looks at me in disbelief. Will I ever slow down?

Probably not.

And especially not now. This year a phenomenon took place, one that has left me astonished, pleased, and incredibly touched. You. You happened. You, and thousands of other people all across the country, read my book, *The 5-Day Miracle Diet*. You found that your life, too, could change for the better, that you, too, had a piece of yourself that wanted so badly to be thin, energetic, and proud. You discovered, firsthand, like me, that with good blood sugar your physiological cravings disappear—and along with them, the mid-afternoon slump, the blahs, the fatigue, the depression, and the irritability that have very possibly plagued you your entire life.

I knew my diet plan worked. I'd seen the proof in myself and in the clients who have come to see me over the years. But what completely surprised me, what I didn't expect, was the number—and the heartfelt depth—of the reactions I received.

Suddenly there were thousands of people hearing me, asking me questions, running out and buying my book, wanting to talk to me, needing to talk to me, and thanking me. Yes, thanking me for the changes that have occurred in their lives since they began the 5-Day Miracle Diet. Wow!

Whenever I got butterflies in my stomach—before every television show, every radio spot, every interview, and every live appearance during my tour—I thought of you. And I was completely and utterly overwhelmed with love, gratitude, and confidence.

I learned so much from all of you!

Until I went off on my first book tour, I have to admit I felt very concerned about publishing my diet. It was my "baby," my basic philosophy, the lifestyle I passionately believe in. I was overprotective, afraid to let my "child" out the door and into the world.

Happily, all went well. You, thousands and thousands of you, have shared my vision. Indeed, many of you have already begun your own 5-Day Miracle Diet, planning your meals, timing your hard chews, and finding, incredibly enough, that the control you have over your food permeates every aspect of your life!

The letters and phone calls I have received since my book was published have confirmed this. Just like my clients who have come into my office, people all over the United States and Canada have said the same exact thing. They've told me that they've tried every other diet to no avail. But, thanks to my diet plan, they have, at last, found something they could call their own—and lose weight, too.

The phenomenon they are experiencing goes far beyond the 5-Day Miracle Diet. It's called empowerment, and it is heady stuff—not to mention incredibly simple: By the one simple act of controlling your foods, you control your blood sugar...and your life.

Perhaps you, too, have already read *The 5-Day Miracle Diet*. Or perhaps you've just sat down to start the first page. Whatever it is, the pieces may not yet feel complete. Something is missing. You want more, something "extra" to help you understand, to guide you through the next few months. You wish you had a personal guide to "take you by the hand" and help you through the difficult times—and applaud you during your triumphs.

That's where *The 5-Day Miracle Diet Companion* comes in.

I specifically designed this book to be an accompaniment to my program, outlined in detail in *The 5-Day Miracle Diet*.

This companion is a motivational tool, created to help you stick to the basic Puhn principles, to understand your *fathead* issues, to keep you writing down the foods you eat for your own edification. And at the same time, you'll learn some fascinating facts about a variety of food-related subjects. You'll find insights on fat, on fish, and on hard chews. You'll find inspiring quotes and sayings to keep you going strong and your mind focused. You'll find mini-quizzes and bon mots to make you laugh—and stick with it. You'll also discover amazing facts about dieting through the ages that make today's world amazingly easy to deal with. And amidst this lively banter, you'll also find ways to stay on the right track—with the help of an actual journal, a weekly assessment page, and a "Month in the Country of the 5-Day Miracle Diet," where you'll find places to record your weight loss, your reduced inches, and the exciting things that have happened—and will happen—in your life since you began the diet!

And, saving the best for last, there are close to forty recipes here that fit perfectly into the 5-Day Miracle Diet. There are fish and chicken dishes, a succulent lamb entrée, a pasta dish, soups, salads and salad dressings, and vegetable side dishes that are so delicious you'll never go "plain" again. There's even an extra-special "Food You Adore" dessert that is so tempting that even I won't keep it in the house!

It is your book and you should have fun with it. Unlike a library book, this is yours—to write in, to jot down your thoughts in, to draw in, or just plain doodle in. Use it. Embrace it. Even color it in neon pinks and blues!

I hope you will use this book. I urge you to treat it as your personal diary, your guide to a whole new life. And I'll be there, too, every step of the way, cheering you on and sharing your experiences. At the book's end, I'll still be a presence, full of love and happiness, and ready to congratulate you for accomplishing what you set out to do: to begin and stick with the 5-Day Miracle Diet—to begin and stick with a brand-new life.

Enjoy.
Learn.
Relish.
Sample.
And be entertained.

One final note: I'd really like to know what miracles you have had in your life since you began the 5-Day Miracle Diet—and any other thoughts you'd like to share. Please write me and tell what *you* think. Send your notes and letters to me in care of my publishers:

> Ballantine Books
> 201 East 50th Street
> New York, NY 10022

In the meantime, good luck.
And have fun!

> —*Adele Puhn*
> *June 27, 1996*

Here's a sample journal to help you begin...

● ●

Date: *September 25, 1996*

What I ate...for breakfast: *1 oz. turkey, 1 whole-grain bread slice*

What I ate...for my morning hard-chew snacks: *apple, handful of string beans*

What I ate...for lunch: *salad (carrot for hard-chew ribbon), grilled chicken breast-2 oz., 1 small roll.*

What I ate...for my afternoon soft chews: *1 orange*

What I ate...for dinner: *Chinese take out: steamed veggies & 5 oz. tofu, mustard, 1/2 c. steamed brown rice*

How I felt: *only third day, so a little dizzy. Actually yelled at friend at work. But also accomplished a lot more work than I usually do. I sang a song on my way home from work. Keep it up, it's obviously working!*

How I kept moving: *walked to & from office—20 city blocks each way. Used stairs between floors instead of elevators.*

What I drank: *2 big bottles Evian, plus herb tea at desk & before going to sleep. 3 cups coffee (cut down from 5!), drop of milk.*

Did I take my vitamins? *Yes*

*C*ongratulations! You're about to embark on your first month on the 5-Day Miracle Diet. Most probably, these first five days will be the toughest. It might be hard to imagine that when this month is through, you'll be remembering when you couldn't dream of *not* eating that banana or that bagel at breakfast. Or that after-dinner snack—you know, that chocolatey thing you couldn't watch *ER* without chowing down on.

I'm not saying it won't be a month of ups and downs. And I'm not saying that there still aren't nights when chocolate sounds great. You might be facing your *fathead* issues for the first time in your life—which is difficult indeed. You might even be discovering that, whoops, you're a carbo addict and that pasta might have to become an acquaintance instead of a best friend. But write in your journal, put down all the foods you'll be eating at a steady, timely pace. Jot down your feelings and experiences. On the whole, I'll guarantee you'll be eating healthier and feeling better than you ever have before in your life!

Think about your body. Isn't it exciting to know that it will feel stronger soon? That your skin will glow health? That you are getting an incredible amount of work done without those afternoon slumps? I repeat:

Congratulations are in order! You're about to become a star—in your own life.

Inch-by-Inch

Bust/chest: _____   Upper arms: _____

Wrists: _____   Waist: _____

Abdomen: _____   Hips and buttocks: _____

IN A WORD...

You'll be summing up your monthly experience in one or two words. Use it as your mantra in the month to come. It's easy now that you've made the 5-Day Miracle Diet yours to keep! Here's one of my favorites:

I'm on my way—at last!

What's your good word?

_____

Shout it out. You should feel proud!

*T*he next time you take your measurements, have another tape measure handy. Snip off the inches that you lost on the second tape. Keep them in an envelope and watch the envelope get stuffed—not you!

It's all about choices: big choices and little choices.

Having the ability to make those choices is freedom. Make the right ones about your diet, and you'll be free. It's as simple as that!

WEIGHTY ISSUES

Starting weight: _____

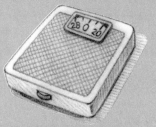

• •

When you need inspiration, look to nature. Animals don't diet.
Have you ever seen a fat deer? And contemplating the great
outdoors does wonders for your psyche, too!

• •

A WEEK'S "POCKETFUL OF MIRACLES"

Welcome to the world of miracles, a place that will exist in you, thanks to the 5-Day Miracle Diet. This sidebar will become an old friend before our six months together are spent, and I hope it will continue to be with you long after our journey together is through.

This is where you'll put those wonderful observations that will occur as you start living on the 5-Day Miracle Diet. Perhaps you'll jot down the way your body feels, strong and vital. Perhaps you'll want to express your amazement at your newfound energy and zest for life. Or maybe you'll simply be pleased to be on an even keel for the first time in your life.

Your weekly miracle can be about your body, your soul, your emotions, or the way you now look at food—anything that you feel is a major accomplishment in your life.

For this first week, write down what you expect to accomplish within these six months on my diet plan. We'll come back to it at the very last week to see if your hope has been realized.

Here's an example from a man who'd been to see me for about two months:

• *What do I want from this diet? Well, some peace of mind would be nice. Yes, a sense of calm that follows me throughout the day.*

Now it's your turn:_____

_____

_____

"I can tell you how wonderful you are going to feel once you're in good blood sugar. But it doesn't matter. You won't be able to really see it for yourself until you experience it. And then, wow!"

—*The Daily Adele Dose*

• •

Date:

What I ate...for breakfast: _____

_____

_____

What I ate...for my morning hard-chew snacks: _____

_____

What I ate...for lunch: _____

_____

_____

_____

What I ate...for my afternoon soft chews: _____

What I ate...for dinner: _____

_____

_____

_____

How I felt: _____

_____

_____

How I kept moving: _____

_____

_____

What I drank: _____

_____

Did I smile more at other people today—because I wanted to?

_____

A THOUGHTFUL PAUSE

Renew your motivation with a little (creative) visual aid. A calm, peaceful body will resist the need to eat. How to get to that center? When you awaken in the morning, take a few moments to meditate before hopping out of bed. Here's what to do:

1. Press your snooze alarm for ten more minutes (so you won't go back to sleep!).
2. Take a deep breath in. Slowly exhale.
3. Repeat three times.
4. Visualize a "safe" haven in your mind—a forest, a meadow, or a seashore—a place that makes you feel safe, calm, and at peace.
5. Imagine yourself in this wonderful place.
6. Tell yourself, "I am a special, loving person."
7. Tell yourself, "I deserve to treat my body with respect."
8. Repeat these thoughts three times.
9. Breathe deeply once again. Exhale.
10. Open your eyes and begin your day, refreshed and ready to be healthy!

Centuries Ahead of His Time

"It is part of a wise man to feed himself with moderate pleasant food and drink."

—The philosopher Spinoza (1632–1677)

"Are you ready to feel absolutely fabulous? Let's go!"
                                        —The Daily Adele Dose

• •

Date:

What I ate...for breakfast: _____
_____
_____

What I ate...for my morning hard-chew snacks: _____
_____

What I ate...for lunch: _____
_____
_____
_____

What I ate...for my afternoon soft chews: _____

What I ate...for dinner: _____
_____
_____
_____

How I felt: _____
_____
_____

How I kept moving: _____
_____
_____

What I drank: _____
_____

Did I try a different starch today, instead of the typical pasta/rice/
potato? _____

PAUL AND THE SINGING TELEGRAM

Paul looked so sad when he first came to see me. He had no spirit, he told me, no zest for life. "And I'm an actor," he continued. "I have to be larger than life!"

Paul was only about fifteen pounds too heavy for his frame, but it was enough for him to be rejected for television commercials, TV roles, the movies—any spot where young sexy men were wanted.

"Restaurants don't even want me," he groaned. "The only work I can get is in a gorilla suit singing 'Happy Birthday' to someone who opens the door with a stunned look on his face."

I smiled. I knew that Paul was in bad blood sugar and that it was this imbalance that was talking. I didn't say anything. I simply put Paul on the 5-Day Miracle Diet and asked him to come to see me next week. When he came back, he was smiling, his grin showing off every one of his bright white teeth.

"So, Paul," I said, "how do you feel?"

"Great!" he replied. "I feel so good I can't tell you. And I got my first role!"

Paul had decided that the wonderful feeling he had was much more important than the fifteen pounds he wanted to lose. During the week, as his blood sugar became balanced, his thinking became clearer. "I was looking for the wrong roles," he said. "I'm a character actor, and character actors can weigh fifteen pounds more than leading men. It's okay!"

Today, Paul is earning his living by playing a role. He's a well-respected actor on a popular television drama. And by the way, he's lost a total of twenty pounds, not fifteen!

"On my special 5-Day Miracle Diet plan, this will become the way you eat. The old will be the exception— not the rule."

—*The Daily Adele Dose*

● ●

Date: _____

What I ate...for breakfast: _____
_____
_____

What I ate...for my morning hard-chew snacks: _____
_____

What I ate...for lunch: _____
_____
_____
_____

What I ate...for my afternoon soft chews: _____

What I ate...for dinner: _____
_____
_____
_____

How I felt: _____
_____
_____

How I kept moving: _____
_____
_____

What I drank: _____
_____

Did I skip the roll at lunch today because I simply didn't want it (even though I knew I could have it)? _____

YOU CAN'T GO HOME AGAIN

Here's some "nonfood" for thought: Who would want to fit into that pair of jeans from high school anyway? Most probably, they are outmoded bell-bottoms or pencil-thin, can't-breathe, scratchy designer denims or baggy-in-the-knees-and-stomach jeans that would make even Keanu Reeves look fat!

Be wary of this kind of "denim lemon." You'll be setting yourself up to fail. Think about it: All that time and energy to finally, at last, put on something that makes you look (to put it nicely) silly!

Instead, get thee to a store and go for a new pair of stylish jeans that make you look smashing—right now!

"What I find so amazing about this diet is how simple it is. I mean, I can live on this plan. I can really live on it—wherever I am!"

—A fifty-year-old businessman who has already lost twenty-two pounds on the 5-Day Miracle Diet

"You need to think about foods in the beginning because you are changing old habits into new—healthier and more vital—ones!"

—The Daily Adele Dose

• •

Date:

What I ate...for breakfast: _____

_____

_____

What I ate...for my morning hard-chew snacks: _____

_____

What I ate...for lunch: _____

_____

_____

_____

What I ate...for my afternoon soft chews: _____

What I ate...for dinner: _____

_____

_____

_____

How I felt: _____

_____

_____

How I kept moving: _____

_____

_____

What I drank: _____

_____

Did I try drinking unsweetened herb tea today instead of coffee? _____

MIRACLE DIET WARNING: Chocolate is a fact of food life. As a service to all of you who feel you're going straight to chocolate hell if you so much as look at a morsel, I've compiled this list. But please: This is not an ad to entice you to eat some chocolate. I repeat. Chocolate is, and always will be, a "Food You Adore"—an "Extra"!!!

CHOCOLATE FACTS:
Food for the Soul, "Food You Adore"

Chocolate is one of those buzzwords. It puts fear in the minds of people who are trying to lose weight (and maybe one or two Puritans). And to be fair, it's true that choosing chocolate (in any form) as your "Food You Adore" will cause your blood sugar to wobble for a day or two. But many people are willing to "walk the wobble." Now, I'm not advocating chocolate as an every-week "Food You Adore" treat, but if you truly love chocolate (and I know I do!), it's nice to know that you haven't destroyed all your good efforts if you partake. In fact, there's a lot worse out there! To reassure you that a chocolate "Extra" does not a binge make, here are some fat-scinating facts about our "forbidden fruit":

✔ Chocolate has less caffeine than a cup of coffee—less than 7 mg per ounce!

✔ A chocolate kiss has a mere 23 calories.

✔ One large chocolate marshmallow only has 19 calories.

✔ Studies have found no "solid chocolate" evidence that chocolate makes your skin break out.

✔ Chocolate is not the cause of cavities—sugar is. But since sugar is one of the ingredients that makes up the chocolate we know and love, you'll be getting a taste of "refined sweet" with every bite. It's why chocolate is considered a "Food You Adore" choice instead of a staple.

✔ Chocolate and cholesterol don't mix. The cocoa bean is a plant (which has 0 cholesterol). Even after the "good stuff," like milk solids and butter, have been added, a chunk of chocolate has less than 8 mg of cholesterol in every 1-ounce bite.

✔ Chocolate stimulates the release of endorphins in the brain, the same chemicals that make you feel lightheaded, exhilarated, and exuberant when you're in love!

"Once you've been on my program for five days, the fun begins. You get to eat the 'Food You Adore' once or twice a week!"

—*The Daily Adele Dose*

• •

Date:

What I ate...for breakfast: _____
_____
_____

What I ate...for my morning hard-chew snacks: _____
_____

What I ate...for lunch:_____
_____
_____
_____

What I ate...for my afternoon soft chews: _____

What I ate...for dinner:_____
_____
_____
_____

How I felt: _____
_____
_____

How I kept moving: _____
_____
_____

What I drank: _____
_____

Did I do one or two—or three—more things than I thought I could, thanks to my extra energy? _____

LET THE RECIPES BEGIN....

You'll soon come across some of the fabulous recipes I've created in my kitchen with the help of two award-winning chefs. I hope you enjoy every single bite of these low-calorie, nutritious entrées, side dishes, soups, and salads, and even a fantastic dessert!

There's only one rule: Keep a running tab on your daily allotments, especially the amount of oil you can have each day on the 5-Day Miracle Diet.

RECIPE GUIDE

"Keep your food and snacks simple in the beginning. That way it will be easy to stick to my diet!"

—The Daily Adele Dose

• •

Date:

What I ate...for breakfast: _____

_____

What I ate...for my morning hard-chew snacks: _____

_____

What I ate...for lunch: _____

_____

_____

What I ate...for my afternoon soft chews: _____

What I ate...for dinner: _____

_____

_____

_____

How I felt: _____

_____

_____

How I kept moving: _____

_____

_____

What I drank: _____

_____

Did I continue to keep track of my foods and my emotions in my diary? _____

SUMMER SHRIMP

I call this dish a "gift from the sea." It is so easy to prepare that I am thankful every time I make it for company. It is a combination of both cold and hot, and is also versatile and convenient. You can make this with either shrimp or calamari, whatever looks best at the seafood counter. And whichever you choose, you'll enjoy every savory bite of this unusual salad.

What you'll need:

24 ounces medium to large shrimp (21 to 25 shrimp per pound), peeled, cleaned, and deveined, or 24 ounces calamari
32 ounces string beans
15 chopped basil leaves
 3 tablespoons chopped parsley
 6 tablespoons extra-virgin olive oil
1½ tablespoons fresh oregano or ¾ teaspoon dry
   Salt and pepper to taste
   Plum (Roma) tomatoes, for garnish

What you'll do:

Steam the shrimp for 3 minutes. Or boil the calamari for 1 hour in lightly salted water. Slice the calamari very thin.

Steam the string beans for 2 minutes and cut them in half.

Mix all the ingredients well in a large bowl. Place mixture in a flat dish and surround the salad with thin slices of tomato.

Serve immediately.

Serves 4 (male-sized) portions. Women: Spoon about 2 ounces fish mixture into a plastic container. Cover and place in fridge to eat for breakfast or add to lunch or dinner the next day. Both men and women: Don't forget to add the oil toward your daily fat allotment.

MIRACLE DIET CHEF'S HINT: The numbers "21/25" that you see for the shrimp ingredient is a way to measure the size you'll need—so you won't eat too many or too little on the 5-Day Miracle Diet. The size is based on the amount of shrimp you'd need per pound. In other words, you'd need 21 to 25 shrimp to make a pound in this recipe—which, translated, means you'll need large shrimp. If you had to have approximately 40 shrimp to make a pound, you'd be using medium shrimp. Size 10 shrimp would be jumbo size.

"By starting the 5-Day Miracle Diet, you have decided to do something positive about your life. You have made the choice to be healthy and live a full and vital life!"

—*The Daily Adele Dose*

• •

Date:

What I ate...for breakfast: _____
_____
_____

What I ate...for my morning hard-chew snacks: _____
_____

What I ate...for lunch: _____
_____
_____
_____

What I ate...for my afternoon soft chews: _____

What I ate...for dinner: _____
_____
_____
_____

How I felt: _____
_____
_____

How I kept moving: _____
_____
_____

What I drank: _____
_____

Did I order exactly *what I wanted at the restaurant tonight?*
_____

WEIGHTY ISSUES

Last week's weight: _____

Pounds lost: _____

New weight: _____

Don't forget those lost ounces and half pounds. They add up!

• •

There are lessons everywhere. Have you ever heard a flight attendant tell a group of passengers to put on their own oxygen masks before helping others? You have to take care of yourself—your body and your health— before you can take on the world! The 5-Day Miracle Diet will help you help others, too!

• •

A WEEK'S "POCKETFUL OF MIRACLES"

Congratulations! You've just completed your first week on the 5-Day Miracle Diet. And your body chemistry thanks you for healthy eating, positive, calm energy, and strong, flexible fat-burning movement.

Take a moment to think about the wonderful "miracles" this diet has brought to your life. Write them down. Better yet, post them on your mirror!

Here's one to get you started—a "miracle" a client told me about with a great big grin on his face:
•*I walked up the subway stairs without puffing when I reached the top. A first!*

Now it's your turn: _____

_____

_____

"Imagine: No more cravings. No more fatigue. No more mood swings. And all it takes is five days to get you going!"

—*The Daily Adele Dose*

• •

Date:

What I ate...for breakfast: _____
_____
_____

What I ate...for my morning hard-chew snacks: _____
_____

What I ate...for lunch:_____
_____
_____
_____

What I ate...for my afternoon soft chews: _____

What I ate...for dinner:_____
_____
_____
_____

How I felt: _____
_____
_____

How I kept moving: _____
_____
_____

What I drank: _____
_____

Did I eat the appropriate amounts of food at meals?
_____

If You Are Bored, Don't Be Boring!

There's more to life than steamed white rice. In fact, there are 15,000 different types of rice available in the world today!

FORGET THE SCALE

Losing weight is a process, like life itself. And it has nothing to do with the numbers on the scale. Some days you'll feel thinner just because you're feeling good about yourself. Other days, despite a decent weight loss, you'll feel fat and disgusting because something happened to make you feel bad about yourself. (A typical *fathead* saboteur!)

The best way to stop the confusion and its possible sabotage: Concentrate on the inside—the way you feel, the energy you have, the vitality and strength that surge through you. With positive thinking and healthful growth, your actual weight will lose its importance, in your mind, body, and soul!

"Give me five days and I will change your life!"

—*The Daily Adele Dose*

• •

Date:

What I ate...for breakfast: _____
_____
_____

What I ate...for my morning hard-chew snacks: _____
_____

What I ate...for lunch: _____
_____
_____
_____

What I ate...for my afternoon soft chews: _____

What I ate...for dinner: _____
_____
_____
_____

How I felt: _____
_____
_____

How I kept moving: _____
_____
_____

What I drank: _____
_____

Did I eat enough vegetables with my protein at lunch?
_____

BRUSSELS SPROUTS PROVENÇALE

Brussels sprouts are one of those misunderstood vege-tables. People know they're good for them, but they don't have a clue how to cook them so they taste good. Well, your confusion is at an end. When I first tasted this elegant side dish, I knew I had a Brussels sprouts recipe for life. I hope you enjoy it as much as I do!

What you'll need:

16 ounces Brussels sprouts, cleaned and cut in half lengthwise
 1 tablespoon extra-virgin olive oil
 1 tablespoon chopped scallions
 2 tablespoons chopped red bell pepper
 2 tablespoons chopped onions
 1 tablespoon chopped basil
 1 tablespoon chopped leeks, green part only
½ cup chopped very ripe plum (Roma) tomatoes
 2 cups low-fat chicken broth
    Salt and pepper to taste
    Red pepper slices, for garnish
    Asparagus tips, boiled, for garnish

What you'll do:

Steam the Brussels sprouts for 2 minutes. Set aside.

Heat the oil in a large nonstick skillet. Add the scallions, red bell pepper, onions, basil, and leeks and sauté until golden.

Add tomatoes and chicken broth. Bring to a boil and boil for one minute. Remove from heat and add salt and pepper to taste.

Put the mixture in a blender or food processor. Blend for one minute. Pour ingredients into an 8-quart saucepan. Add the Brussels sprouts, cover, and simmer for 10 minutes.

Serve Brussels sprouts on a flat dish, decorated with sliced red peppers and boiled asparagus tips.

Serves 4. Don't forget to add the oil to your fat allotment for the day.

"Think about it. You're starting a whole new way of being, a new way of life. Isn't it exciting!"

—*The Daily Adele Dose*

• •

Date:

What I ate...for breakfast: _____

_____

_____

What I ate...for my morning hard-chew snacks: _____

_____

What I ate...for lunch: _____

_____

_____

_____

What I ate...for my afternoon soft chews: _____

What I ate...for dinner: _____

_____

_____

_____

How I felt: _____

_____

_____

How I kept moving: _____

_____

_____

What I drank: _____

_____

Did I get in some cardiovascular exercise? _____

THE WOMAN AND THE BLACK LEGGINGS

When Bonnee first came to see me, she was only slightly over-weight, about fifteen pounds to be exact. But those fifteen pounds were like fifty on someone else: She'd look in the mirror and see a "fat" body.

I looked at Bonnee that first week and I saw a beautiful, poised, and capable-looking woman. She appeared every bit the empowered woman . . . a graphic artist by day, a mother of three at night. She was stylishly dressed in leggings and a striking lemon-yellow silk blouse.

But the dual roles were getting to her, I could tell. There were rings around her eyes, and she hated to leave her children in the morning.

Before we began to discuss her life, I knew that Bonnee had to get into good blood sugar. That first week, I put her on the 5-Day Miracle Diet and simply asked her to do the best she could.

Bonnee came back the next week and had lost one pound, but she was still full of pain. "That's all? One pound? Forget it! I'm hopeless!" she exclaimed, ready to walk out the door for good.

I told her to wait. I looked at her journal. Sure enough, there were several hard chews missing. There was an evening out with two glasses of wine. There was even a dinner that hadn't been written down.

This went on for two more weeks. I asked her directly if perhaps she didn't want to lose weight.

That startled her—and jolted her into thinking about her *fathead* issues. "I want to lose weight, Adele, but I don't want to open any doors. I can't leave my job, but I hate what it's doing to me emotion-ally. I feel I'm not there for my kids. That's why I wear these." Bonnee stood up and showed me her leggings, those wonderful black stretchy pants that "grow" with you. "As long as my leggings fit me, I feel I don't have to do anything. I don't have to look at my life. Silly, huh?"

No, not silly at all, I assured her. I told her that together we could work out her problems. Three months later, Bonnee is working at home two days a week—a perfect solution to her juggling act. The message? Stay with your 5-Day Miracle Diet. Who knows what solu-tions you'll find to your seemingly insurmountable problems!

> *"It's happening, isn't it? Your first thought in the morning isn't about food!"*
>
> —*The Daily Adele Dose*

● ●

Date:

What I ate...for breakfast: _____

_____

What I ate...for my morning hard-chew snacks: _____

_____

What I ate...for lunch: _____

_____

_____

What I ate...for my afternoon soft chews: _____

What I ate...for dinner: _____

_____

_____

How I felt: _____

_____

How I kept moving: _____

_____

What I drank: _____

_____

Did I take enough hard chews to work today, just in case the meeting runs late? _____

DESK SETS

Here are some simple stretches to keep you supple and toned while working at your desk.

1. Take a deep breath. Gently twist your head from side to side, back to front. Repeat five times.

2. Pull off your shoes. (No one will see you.) Turn your ankles to the right, then the left. Repeat for a count of sixty.

3. Take your hands off the computer keyboard. Move them straight out to the side. Take a deep breath and sit up tall, your head held high. Make medium circles in the air, first to the front, then to the left—twenty circles in all.

4. Take another deep breath, and while inhaling, clench your face, your teeth, your hands, your feet, your entire body. Exhale and let go. Repeat twice.

Don't you feel better? And you didn't even have to get up from your chair!

"The 5-Day Miracle Diet is a miracle you make happen!"
                                                    —*The Daily Adele Dose*

• •

Date:

What I ate...for breakfast: _____

_____

_____

What I ate...for my morning hard-chew snacks: _____

_____

What I ate...for lunch: _____

_____

_____

_____

What I ate...for my afternoon soft chews: _____

What I ate...for dinner: _____

_____

_____

_____

How I felt: _____

_____

_____

How I kept moving: _____

_____

_____

What I drank: _____

_____

*Did I take my monthly measurements and write them down
in my journal?* _____

CURB CARBO CONFUSION NOW!

Life isn't always fair, especially when it comes to men and women and their diets. Because of their physiology and body chemistry, men can usually eat more calories and more types of food and still lose weight. On the 5-Day Miracle Diet, men also get the advantage: They can have a starchy carbohydrate every day with an animal protein. Women can only have this combo every other day.

But as with anything else, there's a way around this. Listen up, ladies! If you have a *vegetarian* meal, you, too, can have a starchy carbohydrate every day!

HINTS FROM THE VEGGIE CHEF

Here are some words of wisdom on veggie lore:

• **Buy pre-washed, pre-made salad mixes.** Simply grab a handful of greens for your dinner and tie the remainder up with one of those twist ties. These pre-packs all have at least one-week expiration dates printed on the bag.

• **Buy bulk.** If you have the time and want to save some money, go for the traditional route. Buy your greens unwashed and uncut. Wash and dry cut-up lettuce in a spinner. Keep things simple and convenient by storing greens crisp and dry in a large plastic container with an airtight lid.

"In the real world you don't take a scale to a restaurant. My diet is all about the real world, so use your judgment when you're eating out—and have a good time, too!"
—*The Daily Adele Dose*

• •

Date:

What I ate...for breakfast: _____

_____

What I ate...for my morning hard-chew snacks: _____

_____

What I ate...for lunch: _____

_____

_____

What I ate...for my afternoon soft chews: _____

What I ate...for dinner: _____

_____

_____

How I felt: _____

_____

How I kept moving: _____

_____

What I drank: _____

_____

Did I ask for my sushi made with less rice at the Japanese restaurant?

_____

BEING SELFLESS CAN BE SELF-LESS!

When David came to see me, he was extremely obese—over 300 pounds, in fact. His health was being seriously compromised, and the first thing I needed to do was put him on the 5-Day Miracle Diet.

I knew there had to be a big *fathead* issue behind all this weight, but I also knew that we couldn't tackle it until David's body was in good blood sugar. I encouraged him to call me anytime he had a problem. I needed him to get through those five days so that he would experience what it felt like to be in GBS. I knew the energy, the focus, and the sense of confidence and well-being would go far in helping him to start talking about his *fathead*.

It took several months, but David now "owns" the diet. After he'd taken care of his physiological cravings, he began to write down his feelings. Every time he had a craving, he questioned it. He began to explore his own particular brand of *fathead* that made him want to eat—issues that had begun a long time ago in his childhood home.

David's mother was a self-sacrificing woman, always talking about selfish people who, unlike her, wouldn't do the "right" thing. She lived her life as a martyr, helping others, but doing nothing for herself. David got the message: You are not allowed to think of yourself. You must always think of others first.

His grandmother lived with them as well. This very sick woman became David's responsibility. His mother would demand, "Go upstairs and bring your grandmother her dinner." "Help your grandmother down the stairs." And on and on and on . . .

David did as he was told. After all, he grew up believing that he should take care of others, despite the toll it took on him. But he was angry, too. The fact was, he didn't want to take care of his grandmother all the time. He wanted to have some fun, but he could not deal with the feelings these normal thoughts provoked.

How could he break his mother's heart? Besides, his anger made him feel guilty. He must be a horrible person to even think of having fun!

So David took the only defense he had at his disposal: his weight. He began to eat. And eat. And eat. Soon he couldn't do anything for anybody, including his grandmother. Even better, he didn't have to feel like one of those selfish people his mother was always criticizing. He was simply too fat! David got what he wanted all right, but at a terrible price.

Today, however, David is a changed man. He is able to see that if the opposite of being selfish is self-less, then being selfish can be a very good thing!

"Giving in to temptation makes you human. Learn from these occasions. And call them practice for Real Life!"

—*The Daily Adele Dose*

• •

Date:

What I ate...for breakfast: _____
_____
_____

What I ate...for my morning hard-chew snacks: _____
_____

What I ate...for lunch: _____
_____
_____
_____

What I ate...for my afternoon soft chews: _____

What I ate...for dinner:_____
_____
_____
_____

How I felt: _____
_____
_____

How I kept moving: _____
_____
_____

What I drank: _____
_____

Did I give in to temptation today—and keep going on the diet?
_____

WEEKLY ASSESSMENT

WEIGHTY ISSUES

Last week's weight: _____

Pounds lost: _____

New weight: _____

Don't forget those lost ounces and half pounds. They add up!

• •

Rome wasn't built in a day. Neither can a slimmer, trimmer you! Go slow and steady—you'll see progress that, although it might not launch a whole civilization, will make you feel wonderful for a long, long time!

• •

A WEEK'S "POCKETFUL OF MIRACLES"

This week I'd like to concentrate on breakfast. You know, that meal you usually eat on the run, dashing out the door so you won't be late for work. I think of all the meals on my diet, breakfast is the one that holds the most "miracles."

Think about it. Before you started my program, you probably drank a glass of orange juice. You might have had a plain bagel to complete the meal. Later, at work, when your blood sugar dropped and you needed to eat, you opted for a light yogurt, thinking how virtuous you were. A good positive thought—for about five minutes, until the sugar from all this food "hit" and the cravings began. The result? A fattening lunch—or a miserable, white-knuckled, sacrificing affair. Jot down a breakfast "miracle" you had this week.

Here's one to get you started:

• *Those first five days were tough, no doubt about it. But now? Forget it! I never wake up and smell the coffee!*

Now it's your turn: _____

_____

_____

"My program is specifically designed to work with the body—not against it!"

—*The Daily Adele Dose*

• •

Date:

What I ate...for breakfast: _____

_____

_____

What I ate...for my morning hard-chew snacks: _____

_____

What I ate...for lunch: _____

_____

_____

_____

What I ate...for my afternoon soft chews: _____

What I ate...for dinner: _____

_____

_____

_____

How I felt: _____

_____

_____

How I kept moving: _____

_____

_____

What I drank: _____

_____

Did I wake up with less anxiety and a cleaner head—a first for me?

_____

♦ 33 ♦

CHICKEN SALAD PRIMAVERA

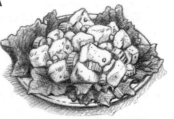

Salads make a delicious, convenient staple for lunch or dinner. Almost any vegetable will do. Mix with greens and some protein and you have a complete meal. This one is particularly satisfying, because it uses vegetables not often used in salad. You can easily make this the night before and bring it to work in a container. Serve with my Tricolore Dressing and your office will be converted into an elegant Italian restaurant!

What you'll need:
- ¾ cup broccoli florets
- ¾ cup asparagus tips
- ½ cup julienne-cut red bell pepper
- 4 skinless, boneless chicken breast halves, about 4 ounces each
- 1 tablespoon extra-virgin olive oil
- 1 tablespoon chopped thyme, or ¼ teaspoon dried
- ¼ cup chopped onion
- 1 tablespoon chopped basil
- Salt and pepper to taste
- 2 cups salad greens made from equal amounts of radicchio, endive, arugula, and sliced tomatoes
- Tricolore Dressing (page 36)

What you'll do:

Steam the broccoli, asparagus, and red bell pepper for 2 minutes. Set aside.

Pound the chicken breasts as flat as possible between two pieces of wax paper.

Heat a large nonstick skillet until water sizzles in its center. Add the oil and chicken and sauté the chicken on each side for 2 minutes.

Remove the chicken from the skillet and slice into julienne strips. Set aside.

Place the steamed vegetables in the skillet. Add the thyme, onion, basil, salt, and pepper and sauté for 2 minutes. Add the chicken and sauté mixture for 1 more minute.

Place the salad ingredients together in a flat dish, mix in the Tricolore Dressing, and pour the hot chicken and vegetables over the salad.

Serves 4. Men: Add 1–2 ounces part-skim mozzarella cheese to salad ingredients. Don't forget to add the oil toward your daily allotment of fat.

"Hard chew does not mean biting into a number-2 pencil! I created the phrase for those foods you need to eat to raise and maintain your good blood sugar levels. And yes, they are harder to chew than other vegetables and fruits!"

—*The Daily Adele Dose*

• •

Date:

What I ate...for breakfast: _____

_____

_____

What I ate...for my morning hard-chew snacks: _____

_____

What I ate...for lunch: _____

_____

_____

_____

What I ate...for my afternoon soft chews: _____

What I ate...for dinner: _____

_____

_____

_____

How I felt: _____

_____

_____

How I kept moving: _____

_____

_____

What I drank: _____

_____

Did I eat my first hard chew within two hours of breakfast? _____

TRICOLORE DRESSING

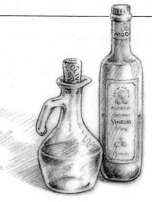

This deliciously spicy vinaigrette is the perfect
accompaniment to a tricolored salad or a field
salad. It goes with any of my entrées, such
as Napa Valley Chicken (page 106) or Filet
Mignon Piquant (page 202), and side
dishes, such as Asparagus Fromage
(page 172) or Endive Étoile (page 70).

What you'll need:
  2 tablespoons Dijon mustard
 ¼ cup red wine vinegar
  1 tablespoon balsamic vinegar
 ¼ cup extra-virgin olive oil
    Pinch of minced garlic
    Pinch of fresh or dried oregano
    Salt and pepper to taste

What you'll do:
   In a small bowl, mix the mustard and the two vinegars together with a
whisk. Add the oil slowly, mixing gently with the whisk as you go. Add
the garlic, oregano, salt, and pepper and mix until well blended.

Serves 4. Don't forget to add the dressing to your daily allotment of fat.

"There's no doubt about it: This diet is unique! Better yet, it works!"

— *The Daily Adele Dose*

• •

Date:

What I ate...for breakfast: _____

_____

What I ate...for my morning hard-chew snacks: _____

_____

What I ate...for lunch: _____

_____

_____

What I ate...for my afternoon soft chews: _____

What I ate...for dinner: _____

_____

_____

How I felt: _____

_____

How I kept moving: _____

_____

What I drank: _____

_____

Did I eat the right combinations and textures of food today? _____

NOT SO CHICKEN LITTLE

One of the biggest fast-food crazes today is chicken take-out shops. From KFC (a.k.a., in "old-fashioned" vernacular, Kentucky Fried Chicken) to Boston Chicken, rotisserie poultry is all the rage.

These stores do sell some delicious items, and on the surface, everything is "lookin' good"—and lean. But looks can be deceiving, even if you're not ordering the deep-fried stuff.

Rotisserie chicken is still brushed with oil or butter; the skin is still made up of almost 100 percent fat. The side potato and veggie dishes are usually coated in sauce. Even the salads are already tossed with huge amounts of dressing.

The best way to order: Let someone else go up to the display. You don't need to watch the chickens turn on their spits. It can be enough to wake the sleepiest *fathead*.

If you must face the counter, your best bet is to ask the clerk to take the skin off before packing it up. Go for the steamed vegetables, the plain baked potatoes, and the beans. Ask for salad without dressing, and once you get home, use one of the three fabulous dressing recipes you'll find in this book.

You might be feeling worried that you'll miss this "great" food, but you won't. When you're in good blood sugar, you're not going to crave. And if you so choose, ask the clerk to "give you some skin" and make this a night for "Food You Adore."

"You don't have to be perfect. No one is. It's boring. Just be fine. And be yourself!"

—The Daily Adele Dose

● ●

Date:

What I ate...for breakfast: _____
_____
_____

What I ate...for my morning hard-chew snacks: _____
_____

What I ate...for lunch: _____
_____
_____
_____

What I ate...for my afternoon soft chews: _____

What I ate...for dinner:_____
_____
_____
_____

How I felt: _____
_____
_____

How I kept moving: _____
_____
_____

What I drank: _____
_____

*Did I write in my food diary today?*_____

TURN THAT FROWN UPSIDE DOWN

I remember the afternoon Lindsay, a longtime client, made her confession: "When I first came to see you, Adele, I was furious, red-hot angry. At myself, for gaining so much weight, and at you, because I had to make an appointment to see you." Lindsay had laughed and clapped her hands together. "But now I'm happy with the two of us!"

I had smiled. "Of course you are! You are living your life—and loving it!"

I had been so pleased to see Lindsay's new empowerment. I hadn't been surprised to hear about the anger, either—although the confession did seem strange coming from one of the gentlest and kindest people I'd ever met.

Lindsay had gained weight after she had her baby. She'd never lost her thirty "pregnancy pounds." I had put her on the 5-Day Miracle Diet and she, almost immediately, began to lose weight. In fact, she had begun to feel terrific, better than she ever had in her life!

Lindsay and I had worked together for a few months before that afternoon epiphany. I had watched her progress and her burgeoning self-knowledge. A strange thing had happened: As she'd shed those excess pounds, she'd also shed her anger. She had a new feeling, something unfamiliar but wonderful: happiness.

"When you're in low blood sugar and you have a fierce food craving, it's your body's ventriloquist talking. You're just a puppet, and bad blood sugar is pulling your strings!"

—*The Daily Adele Dose*

• •

Date:

What I ate...for breakfast: _____

_____

What I ate...for my morning hard-chew snacks: _____

_____

What I ate...for lunch: _____

_____

_____

What I ate...for my afternoon soft chews: _____

What I ate...for dinner: _____

_____

_____

How I felt: _____

_____

_____

How I kept moving: _____

_____

_____

What I drank: _____

_____

Did I hear a call from a fathead—*and head it off at the pass?*

_____

AND NOW A BRIEF WORD FROM OUR FOOD EXPERTS...

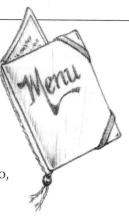

Sometimes I forget which came first: the delicious recipes or the lovely ambience. All I know is that I've been going to Restaurant Navona for years now. Owner and manager Giorgio Meriggi calls it Italian, but it serves food with a continental flair. Once a year, he and his partners, Pasquale Cervere and Tony D'Arcangelo, travel to Italy, Switzerland, France, and Belgium, tasting new foods and experimenting with light sauces and dressings.

Master Chef Roberto Calabrese, who oversees the kitchen in Giorgio's other restaurant, Stresa, and Chef 2000 award recipient Chef Ella Aocca of Restaurant Navona worked with me to make the recipes you've been discovering within the pages of this book. The chefs concentrated their talents on the light recipes which are a staple at both restaurants—where most of their diners are weight-conscious. The result? The scrumptious, unusual, and easy-to-prepare dishes you will, hopefully, soon enjoy first-hand!

Restaurant Navona, now a landmark in Great Neck, New York, began in the minds of Giorgio and Pasquale when they worked at Tre Scalini in Manhattan—which was named after the famous Tre Scalini in the Piazza Navona in Rome. The best table in the New York restaurant was one under a beautiful painting of the Piazza Navona. People would actually wait to be seated there.

When Giorgio and his partners had the opportunity to open their own restaurant, they gave it a name that would evoke the famous piazza and the popular painting—hoping their restaurant, too, would be a place where people would want to sit... and eat!

"Once you're in good blood sugar and you make choices that work for you, you 'own' the diet. No one can ever take it away!"

—*The Daily Adele Dose*

• •

Date:

What I ate...for breakfast: _____
_____
_____

What I ate...for my morning hard-chew snacks: _____
_____

What I ate...for lunch: _____
_____
_____
_____

What I ate...for my afternoon soft chews: _____

What I ate...for dinner: _____
_____
_____
_____

How I felt: _____
_____
_____

How I kept moving: _____
_____
_____

What I drank: _____
_____

Did I eat a timed soft chew this afternoon? _____

A HOME-ALONE CHECKLIST

Friday night couldn't come fast enough. You had been counting the days for this weekend, because at last you had no obligations, no plans, no nothing. You were going to spend the weekend with a good book, a few good videos, and your cat at your side. Maybe you wouldn't even get dressed!

It's all planned down to the minute. You've even gone to the store and bought some 5-Day Miracle Diet staples. You're ready and willing to rest!

But wait...it's nine o'clock in the evening and you're getting bored. Instead of luxuriating in your privacy, you feel lonely. The frozen pizza from last week is saying hello from the freezer. The pretzels in the unopened bag are shaking and dancing. Even the loaf of whole-grain bread is pounding at the bread door. Yikes! It's a cacophony of food sounds, all beckoning you to eat. What are you going to do? Simple. You:

1. Put some soothing oil in your tub and take a long, peaceful bath.

2. Call a long-distance friend you haven't spoken to in a few months.

3. Slowly eat your Chinese take-out steamed vegetables and rice, savoring each bite in your chopsticks, while you watch a video.

4. Take the frozen pizza and the pretzels and carry them to the garbage. All gone!

5. Eat an apple while you watch the second video.

6. Give yourself a facial.

7. Do 300 sit-ups and 300 push-ups while the video rolls on.

8. Trim your hair.

9. Go to sleep! Ahh...what a relaxing night.

*"The 5-Day Miracle Diet is all about living with food—
not living without it!"*

—The Daily Adele Dose

• •

Date:

What I ate...for breakfast: _____

_____

_____

What I ate...for my morning hard-chew snacks: _____

_____

What I ate...for lunch: _____

_____

_____

_____

What I ate...for my afternoon soft chews: _____

What I ate...for dinner: _____

_____

_____

_____

How I felt: _____

_____

_____

How I kept moving: _____

_____

_____

What I drank: _____

_____

*Did I eat a fabulous "Food You Adore" to get rid of the "deprivation
blahs"?*_____

WEEKLY ASSESSMENT

WEIGHTY ISSUES

Last week's weight: _____

Pounds lost: _____

New weight: _____

Don't forget those lost ounces and half pounds. They add up!

• •

Just as happiness comes from within, so do your attitudes about health and diet. They are all tied together: Change one and the others follow suit. Eat healthy on the 5-Day Miracle Diet, and your attitude will change . . . you'll be happy!

• •

A WEEK'S "POCKETFUL OF MIRACLES"

*W*ow, it was a tough week, wasn't it? Well, maybe not this week, but the one before or the one after. A tough week is to be expected at times. And what you have to do is ride it through.

It might sound difficult to stick to your eating plan when your whole world seems to be caving in, but that's what this sidebar is all about: to help you find the motivation to keep on my diet.

Look over your notes from the past weeks. Notice the accumulation of "miracles." They are yours to keep—and embrace. They are designed to make you feel better. After all, another miracle is just a week away!

Here's an example from a man who had certainly seen some rocky roads on his weight-loss journey:

•*The food just didn't do it for me anymore. Not even when I got fired. That's when I started to browse through my journal. I was still miserable, but at least I had my weight loss and my diet!*

Now it's your turn: _____

_____

_____

**"Don't you want to feel better than you ever have in your life?"**

—_**The Daily Adele Dose**_

• •

Date:

What I ate...for breakfast: _____
_____
_____

What I ate...for my morning hard-chew snacks: _____
_____

What I ate...for lunch: _____
_____
_____
_____

What I ate...for my afternoon soft chews: _____

What I ate...for dinner:_____
_____
_____
_____

How I felt: _____
_____
_____

How I kept moving: _____
_____
_____

What I drank: _____
_____

_Did eat the right amounts of protein on my diet today—and with the right meals?_____

TWENTY-VEGETABLE SOUP

Ah! There's nothing like the simmering taste of a hearty soup on a cold night, filling you and nurturing you with good, hot ingredients. This soup is extra-special to me because it manages to be hearty without heavy noodles or pasta. Vegetables are the stars and the chorus line. What makes this dish even more exciting for me is that I eat it all year long. Hot or cold, it makes a delicious repast. And, just in case time and patience are limited, this recipe is easily adaptable. Simply use fewer veggies and call it the Fifteen- or Ten-Vegetable Soup!

What you'll need:

  2 tablespoons extra-virgin olive oil
½ cup chopped onions
½ cup chopped scallions
  5 chopped very ripe plum (Roma) tomatoes
  2 tablespoons chopped basil
  6 cups low-fat chicken broth
  3 cups mixture of the following vegetables, all chopped pea-sized:
     broccoli, carrots, potatoes, zucchini, peas, cabbage, asparagus, cauliflower, bean sprouts, escarole, broccoli rabe, string beans, chicory, Swiss chard, red bell peppers, artichoke, turnip, leeks, radishes, spinach
     Salt and pepper to taste

What you'll do:

   Heat the oil in a large, heavy saucepan and sauté the onions and scallions until golden. Add the tomatoes and basil and simmer for 5 minutes. Add the chicken broth and bring to a boil. Add all the vegetables, bring to a boil, reduce heat, and simmer for 15 minutes, covered. Add salt and pepper to taste.

MIRACLE DIET CHEF'S HINT: This soup keeps for at least 4 days in your refrigerator and longer in the freezer. To serve cold, pour chilled soup, as much as you'll need, into a blender and purée for 2 minutes.

"Put your fathead to bed. When it's time to go to sleep, it's time to go to sleep!"

— *The Daily Adele Dose*

• •

Date:

What I ate...for breakfast: _____
_____
_____

What I ate...for my morning hard-chew snacks: _____
_____

What I ate...for lunch: _____
_____
_____
_____

What I ate...for my afternoon soft chews: _____

What I ate...for dinner: _____
_____
_____
_____

How I felt: _____
_____
_____

How I kept moving: _____
_____
_____

What I drank: _____
_____

Did I take the stairs instead of the elevator today? _____

"SHOOT THE SCALE"!

Not with a gun. But with a quick one-step-two-step action that gets you on and off the scale fast!

Glide those cylinders over the frame if you have a physician's model scale.

Jump off as soon as your number "printout" appears if you have a digital readout scale.

Listen fast, then close your ears if you happen to have one of those voice-activated ones.

Remember: Numbers don't make you a good person. Nor do they make you healthy, wealthy (unless you're Kate Moss), or wise!

The Miracle Behind the 5-Day Miracle

I wanted to share this excerpt from a letter sent to me by a client, a famous college professor who'd recently moved to another city:

The most remarkable thing happened to me this past weekend. My thirtieth class reunion was taking place on Saturday. Usually this would be a sign for me to be really concerned and worried about how I looked, what I could wear, what others would say about my weight. Instead, all I thought about was how excited I was to see my old friends. I couldn't wait!

And the thing is that I've only lost five pounds so far, not enough to make a real difference in what I look like, but eons away from the way I felt at my last reunion.

Thank you for helping me get my life back!

"Every day is another opportunity to stay with the 5-Day Miracle Diet."

—The Daily Adele Dose

• •

Date:

What I ate...for breakfast: _____

_____

What I ate...for my morning hard-chew snacks:_____

_____

What I ate...for lunch:_____

_____

_____

What I ate...for my afternoon soft chews:_____

What I ate...for dinner:_____

_____

_____

How I felt:_____

_____

How I kept moving:_____

_____

What I drank:_____

_____

Did I try a different hard chew today? _____

OUTSTANDING IN HIS FIELD

Lenny had had a problem with his older brother ever since he was a young boy. Whereas he saw himself as Joe Pesci, he saw his brother as George Clooney. He was the nerd; his brother was the class hero. He was the gawky, clumsy guy who couldn't catch a cold; his brother was the athlete who won all the awards.

Lenny looked up to his brother, he loved him. But he couldn't help feeling a bit of sibling rivalry—especially when the girls kept calling and asking for his brother!

Today, Lenny owns a chain of dry-cleaning shops. He has a wife and three kids; he lives in a four-bedroom house in the 'burbs. He's successful and happy. He's still very close to his brother—who became a hot-shot Wall Street lawyer.

But he also weighs in at over 300 pounds. Before he came to me, he tried every diet out there. Nothing. And as his fortieth birthday approached, he had become desperate to change things.

"I feel trapped in this body," he told me at our first meeting. "I'm never going to eat again."

Of course that didn't work. I knew the solution was the 5-Day Miracle Diet. Intellectually, he knew it, too. But still, his fortieth birthday was almost here, and still no weight loss. Despite the fact that he knew what to do, his *fathead* kept getting in the way of his weight loss efforts.

A few sessions later, after reviewing his food journal, I saw the problem in black-and-white: Lenny was simply not eating his hard-chew snacks. Instead of reviewing the journal with him, going over omissions he knew perfectly well were there, I decided to ask him point-blank, "Why don't you want to be thin?"

The question stopped him cold. Suddenly, he knew the answer.

"Ohmigod!" he said after a beat. "If I lose weight, I won't stand out in the crowd. No one will notice me—the way they notice my brother!"

It was a major *fathead* breakthrough. For the first time, Lenny was able to feel his feelings instead of eating them.

By weighing over 300 pounds, he made sure that he *always* stood out in a crowd. On the other hand, he also made sure that he'd never stand out like his brother! Beautifully self-destructive *fathead* logic at its best.

At last, Lenny was free. Not only to lose the weight he so desperately wanted to lose, but free to be himself—not his brother, not some fantasy figure, not a fulfillment of someone else's expectations. He could be Lenny, an outstanding human being in his own right!

> **"If I could eliminate one word out of the English language, it would be self-control."**
>
> —*The Daily Adele Dose*

• •

Date:

What I ate...for breakfast: _____

_____

What I ate...for my morning hard-chew snacks: _____

_____

What I ate...for lunch: _____

_____

_____

What I ate...for my afternoon soft chews: _____

What I ate...for dinner: _____

_____

_____

How I felt: _____

_____

How I kept moving: _____

_____

What I drank: _____

_____

Do I know my target heart-rate zone? _____

Rice di Robella

The award-winning chefs at Restaurant
Navona and Stresa outdid themselves
when they combined creative talents to
conjure up this unusual, healthful, and
scrumptious rice dish. Although it's wonderful with any chicken or lamb dish, it's so
delicious that I'm often tempted to eat it alone for
dinner with a tricolored salad with Tricolore Dressing. This dish is
named after its creators, Roberto and Ella...Robella!

What you'll need:
2   tablespoons extra-virgin olive oil
1/2 cup chopped onion
1/2 cup chopped asparagus
1/2 cup peas
5   cups low-fat chicken broth or stock
2   cups rice, preferably Uncle Ben's Converted white, or brown
3   cups bean sprouts
    Salt and pepper to taste
4   asparagus, uncut, for garnish
16 asparagus tips, 2 inches long

What you'll do:
Heat a nonstick skillet until drops of water sizzle in its center. Add the
oil and onions and sauté until golden brown. Add the chopped asparagus and peas. Mix and set aside.

Bring the chicken broth to a boil in an 8-quart covered saucepan. Add
the rice and cook, covered, for 15 minutes.

Add the bean sprouts and the sautéed mixture. Blend and cook
uncovered for 8 minutes, or until no juice is remaining. Add salt and pepper to taste.

Parboil asparagus stalks and tips for 2 minutes. Arrange a serving dish
with the four asparagus displayed in a star pattern, and add the rice mixture in the middle. Or serve in a family-sized bowl, and place the four
asparagus stalks like trees, standing partway out of the rice. Decorate
with the asparagus tips.

Serves 4. Add the oil and starch to your daily allotments.

"Imagine. No more cravings!"

—The Daily Adele Dose

• •

Date:

What I ate...for breakfast: _____
_____
_____

What I ate...for my morning hard-chew snacks: _____
_____

What I ate...for lunch: _____
_____
_____
_____

What I ate...for my afternoon soft chews: _____

What I ate...for dinner:_____
_____
_____
_____

How I felt: _____
_____
_____

How I kept moving: _____
_____
_____

What I drank: _____
_____

*Did I go over my food lists today to see if there's something on them
I'd like to try?*_____

BANANAS ARE A GROWN-UP'S LOLLIPOPS

Like old-fashioned lollipops, bananas have been ingrained in us because they are a sweet "hit." But unlike candy, they've been touted as perfect diet food—along with bagels and yogurt. In fact, many of us grab a plain bagel or a nonfat yogurt and feel absolutely virtuous. And of course there is that banana we eat in the afternoon when we're in a slump!

These diet die-hards are difficult to give up, especially because you've been consuming them for years while living in low blood sugar. But remember, you've probably been consuming the idea of weight loss for a long time, too—with little success.

The 5-Day Miracle Diet is different. It takes away the food cravings, the afternoon slumps, the fatigue, and the erratic mood swings.

Why? Because it creates and sustains good blood sugar.

How? By the timing, the texture, and the type of food you eat throughout the day—which doesn't leave room (or inclination) for those bagels, nonfat yogurts, and bananas we've been toting around for years.

Consider these foods "extra baggage." They are highly glycemic, converting into sugar much too quickly to keep blood-sugar levels balanced. One bite and poof! They are practically digested before you've even finished every morsel. These foods give you a "hit"—and a craving as soon as they are released in the body.

Afraid to give up your banana? It's the low blood sugar that creates the desperate passion for the food—and it's the subsequent defense *not* to give it up that's talking, not you. You're merely a puppet, playing to your bad-blood-sugar chemistry. But once you've done your first few days on the 5-Day Miracle Diet, you won't miss those bananas. You'll be in good blood sugar and controlling the show.

"After five days, my plan stops sounding like a foreign language. You'll be sure of what you're supposed to do and when you're supposed to do it, thanks to the clear thinking that comes from being in good blood sugar!"

—*The Daily Adele Dose*

• •

Date:

What I ate...for breakfast: _____

_____

_____

What I ate...for my morning hard-chew snacks: _____

_____

What I ate...for lunch: _____

_____

_____

_____

What I ate...for my afternoon soft chews: _____

What I ate...for dinner: _____

_____

_____

_____

How I felt: _____

_____

_____

How I kept moving: _____

_____

_____

What I drank: _____

_____

Did I try a new variety of rice? _____

THE REJECTED BISCOTTI

Essie was a first for me. I'd never tried to help a restaurant owner lose weight, especially not the owner *and* chef of a three-star Italian restaurant in Manhattan!

But it didn't matter what Essie did. What was important was the fact that she wanted to lose weight, that she hated the fifteen pounds of "baggage" she'd been carrying around for six years. "I didn't even carry my ex-husband around as long!" Essie exclaimed in her inimitable style.

I laughed. You couldn't help it with Essie. But with that laughter was a great deal of compassion. Essie had made it the hard way: She had paid her dues for twenty years, working nights and weekends, perfecting dishes long into the night while raising two children solo.

Essie was a small woman. She didn't look capable of handling everything she did. Unfortunately, a lot of what she handled was food—and it seemed to cling to her tiny five-foot frame. "I eat a biscotti, Adele," she complained one afternoon, "a biscotti! Not even something delicious like a cannoli or a perfect risotto, and I gain weight!" She shook her mass of curls. "And I try, I really try to do right by the diet."

Essie sighed. I'd already gone over her food diaries and I saw a missing hard chew here, some berries or an orange after dinner, a pasta lunch. I knew *what* Essie was doing—and I knew that what she did kept the physiological cravings alive. But I didn't know the why, although I had my ideas.

Essie had had it rough when her husband, the co-owner of the restaurant, left her.

Yet Essie persevered. She not only made the restaurant work, she made it a huge success as well. But all that work, all that drive and determination had taken its toll. She was so busy with her restaurant and her children that she never had time to think about dating. She never had to think about what her husband had done. Even better: She never even had time to think about her rage against her ex-husband—or her fear of starting over with someone else. Instead she turned to food.

And because of the restaurant and her line of work, it was the perfect foil!

We talked about this **Double-Indemnity Detractor *fathead*** at length over the next several months. Essie began to recognize the signs of overwhelming emotion: she'd start nibbling a biscotti.

Today, Essie is ten pounds lighter—and she's kept it off. Instead of depriving herself of her own delicious food, she's added some lower-calorie, healthy entrées to her menu.

"Every day you're on the 5-Day Miracle Diet, your body is thanking you!"

—*The Daily Adele Dose*

• •

Date:

What I ate...for breakfast: _____

_____

_____

What I ate...for my morning hard-chew snacks: _____

_____

What I ate...for lunch: _____

_____

_____

_____

What I ate...for my afternoon soft chews: _____

What I ate...for dinner: _____

_____

_____

_____

How I felt: _____

_____

_____

How I kept moving: _____

_____

_____

What I drank: _____

_____

Did I think of trying a different "Food You Adore"—an entrée or appetizer—instead of dessert? _____

*T*ime sure passes quickly when you're having fun. And I sincerely hope that you are having a great deal of fun on the 5-Day Miracle Diet! Now that you've passed those "official" first few weeks, the program has most probably become more and more comfortable, more and more accessible to your lifestyle, easier to live with and easier to do. The miracle in the diet comes from the way you feel, that terrific energy, that newfound zest for life, that fabulous optimism. It also comes from the way you look, the slimmer, trimmer face, the toned body, the "walk that talks."

But as we all know, life is not always a "bowl of hard chews." There will be temptations and psychological cravings.

Don't be discouraged. A cave-in to a craving or a temptation that's become reality can be a real learning experience.

During this next month, jot down those times when you "relapsed." See why they happened and how you handled them. If you can understand the "why," you can "step back" and handle it in a more effective way.

Above all, write in your food journal. You'll see change and growth right there in black-and-white—in only one month.

Imagine what you can do with the rest of your life!

Inch-by-Inch

Bust/chest: _____   Upper arms: _____

Wrists: _____   Waist: _____

Abdomen: _____   Hips and buttocks: _____

IN A WORD...

You'll be summing up your monthly experience in one or two words. Use it as your mantra in the month to come. It's easy now that you've made the 5-Day Miracle Diet yours to keep! Here's one of my favorites:

Life is too important to waste on negative thoughts!

What's your good word?

_____

Shout it out. You should feel proud!

Take a snapshot of yourself at every five-pound loss. Keep the pictures in an album. Date them. You'll see not only the progression of weight loss, but also the figure of a person who stands tall, who's well-groomed, and who has a confident air!

There are always going to be bad days.

Scarlett O'Hara might not have been talking about food when she said, "Tomorrow is another day," but it's true! Stay with it. The good times will come again.

WEEKLY ASSESSMENT

WEIGHTY ISSUES

Last week's weight: _____

Pounds lost: _____

New weight: _____

Don't forget those lost ounces and half pounds. They add up!

• •

The next time you're tempted by a great dessert and you've already eaten your "Food You Adore," think of your brand-new, strong body as dessert—the best one you've ever had in your life!

• •

A WEEK'S "POCKETFUL OF MIRACLES"

*L*ast night, I experienced another miracle. I'd just landed at the airport in a city in the Midwest. I was tired, but exhilarated, too. I was about to begin another round of book tours for *The 5-Day Miracle Diet.*

I looked around for the driver who'd been sent to take me to my hotel. When I found her we started talking, and in the car she told me a moving story. It seemed that her daughter had stopped talking to her months ago. "And then she came home with your book. She started the program four days ago, and, well, it really is a miracle. I guess she's lost weight, but it's more than that. She's talking to me again! She's actually smiling!"

This was my miracle. Here's another one:

• *I was going to write you to tell you how much you changed my life. But after a few more weeks on the diet, I know that's not true. I did it. But you were the best guide I have ever had!*

Now it's your turn: _____

_____

_____

"A good friend is one who never judges you. Why not be a good friend to yourself?"

—The Daily Adele Dose

• •

Date:

What I ate...for breakfast: _____

_____

_____

What I ate...for my morning hard-chew snacks: _____

_____

What I ate...for lunch: _____

_____

_____

_____

What I ate...for my afternoon soft chews: _____

What I ate...for dinner: _____

_____

_____

_____

How I felt: _____

_____

_____

How I kept moving: _____

_____

_____

What I drank: _____

_____

Did I look at myself today in the mirror and not judge the blemish or the double chin? _____

STUFFED POTATO DE LA MER

Like all good food sensualists, I love potatoes! Here's a great way to enjoy them.

What you'll need:

8 10- to 12-ounce red potatoes	6 ounces shrimp, 21/25 size,
¼ cup extra-virgin olive oil	cleaned and cut into 4 pieces
4 ounces chopped scallions	6 ounces salmon, cut into chunks
2 tablespoons chopped shallots	8 chopped plum (Roma) tomatoes
4 ounces chopped onions	¼ cup chopped parsley
6 chopped garlic cloves	¼ cup chopped basil
6 ounces scallops, cut in half	Salt and pepper to taste

What you'll do:

Preheat the oven to 450°F.

Place the potatoes in a baking dish and bake for one hour.

Remove from the oven and let cool. Lower oven to 400°F. (You can also cook potatoes in your microwave oven. Follow the directions for your brand.)

After potatoes have cooked:

Heat a 4-quart saucepan over high heat until a drop of water sizzles in its center. Add the oil, lower the heat to medium, and heat the oil until it sizzles. Add the scallions, shallots, onions, and garlic and sauté until golden.

Add all the seafood and sauté for 2 minutes.

Add the tomatoes, parsley, basil, and ½ cup water. Stir. Cover the saucepan and bring to a boil, then simmer for 8 minutes. Add salt and pepper to taste. Slice off the top of each potato. Scoop out 95 percent of the inside. Fill each potato with equal amounts of seafood mixture and replace the tops of the potatoes. Heat in oven for 4 minutes.

Makes 4 servings, 2 potatoes each (male-sized portions of seafood mixture). Women: Scoop out about 2 ounces seafood mixture and put aside. Store in container in fridge. Eat for lunch or dinner the next day. Don't forget to add the oil toward your daily allotment of fat.

MIRACLE DIET CHEF'S HINT: Don't just throw away the inside of your red potatoes. Store in the fridge. Add herbs to taste and reheat for your own brand of no-fat, low-calorie mashed potatoes! Just don't forget to add them toward your daily allotment of starch.

"When you get into good blood sugar, a remarkable thing happens: You love yourself!"

—*The Daily Adele Dose*

• •

Date:

What I ate...for breakfast: _____

_____

_____

What I ate...for my morning hard-chew snacks: _____

_____

What I ate...for lunch: _____

_____

_____

_____

What I ate...for my afternoon soft chews: _____

What I ate...for dinner: _____

_____

_____

_____

How I felt: _____

_____

_____

How I kept moving: _____

_____

_____

What I drank: _____

_____

Did I take the time to really *read* The 5-Day Miracle Diet *before starting the program?* _____

OVERNIGHT CAMP:
TRAINING GROUNDS FOR THE FUTURE *FATHEAD*

That ubiquitous box of cookies followed me wherever I went as a young girl. I remember that first summer I went off to camp for two weeks. I was so excited: out with the hot, sweltering city and in with the green trees and nature!

Sure, there were those wonderful pines, a lake, and even a little cubbyhole where I could keep my shorts and tops. But nature? It was more like a foodfest! None of us could wait for those care packages from home, those carefully wrapped delights filled with cookies, candy, and more candy. These packages meant our parents cared. Hey, they more than cared. They loved us and missed us! It was the original love connection.

And the canteen! We waited for it to open with more anticipation than mail call. I remember buying two packages of Chuckles and I didn't even like them—it was all they had left.

The worst punishment was not being allowed to go to the canteen. It was the threat our counselors hung over our heads like an imaginary sword. "Don't make your bed—and you won't go to canteen." "If you don't play volleyball, you won't go to canteen." "If you don't fold your clothes, you won't go to canteen." At this point, the "baby" *fatheads* of food/repressed rage, food/fear, food/reward, and food as love began to grow scales, teeth, and a voracious appetite!

Forget nature! Forget starry skies, warm, sunlit days, and canoe rides on the lake. All I wanted was food.

Thanks to my years of education, experience, and evolution, I can appreciate the miracle of nature as much as my miracle diet. But it's easy to see how I became such a food sensualist!

"The food diary is a powerful tool for long-term success. Use it!"

—*The Daily Adele Dose*

• •

Date:

What I ate...for breakfast: _____
_____
_____

What I ate...for my morning hard-chew snacks: _____
_____

What I ate...for lunch: _____
_____
_____
_____

What I ate...for my afternoon soft chews: _____

What I ate...for dinner:_____
_____
_____
_____

How I felt: _____
_____
_____

How I kept moving: _____
_____
_____

What I drank: _____
_____

*Did I eat at the right times today?*_____

THERE'S MORE TO LIFE THAN APPLES AND CARROTS!

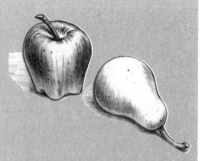

Tired of those typical hard chews? Here are some different ideas that are just as healthy, just as satisfying, and just as capable of creating good blood sugar as the ones you already know:

✔ 1 Chinese pear

✔ 1 handful sliced bok choy. Use the white stalks only; they are crunchy and sweet!

✔ Yellow or waxed string beans

✔ 1 star apple

✔ 1 sapodilla. A pulpy fruit from Central America. Skin looks like potato; pulp is rose-colored and tastes like a sweet pear. (Note: Don't let it become too ripe! You need the hard chew!)

✔ A handful of white Japanese radishes (daikon)

✔ A handful of raw okra, peeled and sliced

✔ Sliced fennel bulbs, raw

"You don't have to conquer the world all in one day. Begin slowly. Build up to exercise as you begin to feel more and more exuberant, more and more alive!"

—*The Daily Adele Dose*

• •

Date:

What I ate…for breakfast: _____

_____

_____

What I ate…for my morning hard-chew snacks: _____

_____

What I ate…for lunch: _____

_____

_____

_____

What I ate…for my afternoon soft chews: _____

What I ate…for dinner: _____

_____

_____

_____

How I felt: _____

_____

_____

How I kept moving: _____

_____

_____

What I drank: _____

_____

Did I think of an exercise, a "Movement You Adore," that I want to give a try? _____

ENDIVE ÉTOILE

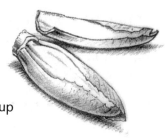

The moon is full, the night is young, and the stars have come out! With this trés French recipe, your side dish has taken on a sparkle. Enjoy this delectable vegetable with one of my chicken or fish entrées and a half cup of couscous. Marvelous!

What you'll need:

8 large endives, cut lengthwise
1 tablespoon extra-virgin olive oil
  Salt and pepper to taste
  Juice of ½ lemon
1 tablespoon balsamic vinegar

What you'll do:

Steam the endives for 4 to 5 minutes in lightly salted water. Drain in a colander.

Heat the oil in a nonstick skillet. Add the endive and sauté each side on medium heat for 2 minutes.

Add salt and pepper, lemon juice, and balsamic vinegar.

Serves 4.

"I'm with you every step of the way, applauding your triumphs and supporting you in tempting times!"

—*The Daily Adele Dose*

• •

Date:

What I ate...for breakfast: _____

_____

_____

What I ate...for my morning hard-chew snacks: _____

_____

What I ate...for lunch: _____

_____

_____

_____

What I ate...for my afternoon soft chews: _____

What I ate...for dinner: _____

_____

_____

_____

How I felt: _____

_____

_____

How I kept moving: _____

_____

_____

What I drank: _____

_____

Did I try putting on an old pair of pants just to see how baggy they are? _____

A Definite Sign of Low Blood Sugar:

"I'm on a seafood diet. I see food and I eat it."

—Anonymous

I'M IN A RECESS STATE OF MIND

We all remember recess, when we rushed out the school doors, ready to play. Recess meant freedom, and as kids, we were going to enjoy every minute of it. Unfortunately, many of us are still in the schoolyard, ready for recess when it comes to vacations and holidays. A "Recess State of Mind" is the saboteur that means forgetting to eat right, forgetting good blood sugar, forgetting you ever heard about the 5-Day Miracle Diet.

I'm not trying to be the "stern principal" here. But I know from personal experience that it is much nicer to go on vacation without the sluggish feeling, to be able to visit museums and tour castles without experiencing that mid-afternoon slump. Enjoy yourself. Enjoy your food. Just don't forget the basics of the program. Bring along the carrots and the green beans on the plane.

"Give me five days and I will give you the rest of your life!"

—*The Daily Adele Dose*

• •

Date:

What I ate...for breakfast: _____
_____
_____

What I ate...for my morning hard-chew snacks: _____
_____

What I ate...for lunch: _____
_____
_____
_____

What I ate...for my afternoon soft chews: _____

What I ate...for dinner: _____
_____
_____
_____

How I felt: _____
_____
_____

How I kept moving: _____
_____
_____

What I drank: _____
_____

*Did I speak up in a restaurant today?*_____

ALL THE WAY HOME, OR, "RECESS": AT PLAY IN FOUR ACTS

There was a whole world in that box of cookies I was born in, a world rich in smells and sights and color found only on the Lower East Side.

And most of that sensory experience centered on food.

It always started on Friday afternoon, right after school. As soon as the school bell rang, my girlfriend and I would run outdoors, our allowance money, doled out on Thursday night, burning a hole in our pockets. There, right outside on the pavement, stood the first food stop: the sweet-potato man and his cart. We'd give him our nickels, and in return receive hot, buttered sweet potatoes on a stick, ready to eat like a Popsicle.

We'd gobble down the potatoes as we continued to walk home, knowing full well that less than two blocks away was the spice stand, a tiny alcove between buildings where a man sold packages of spices and the best pickles in the world. The pickles bobbed in big, brown barrels. We would reach in and select the juiciest, fattest, and most garlicky pickles we could find. And all the while the spice man would yell at us, "Are you done yet? You're holding up the works!" He'd shake his head as, our decision finally made, we paid for our pickles. We held them in the piece of wax paper that contained the juices as we ate.

"Darn kids!" he'd swear under his breath as we left the alcove. But I never really thought he was angry. It was just part of our Friday afternoons, just another food ritual come into play.

We weren't done yet. There was still money in our pockets and miles of food to consume. Just one more street and there was the next "food emporium," shouting out its wares by its prominence in the middle of the block—and the delicious scent that filled the air. Ah, the bakery.

Inside, the smells were intoxicatingly warm and lush. Raisin bread and rugelach were our favorites. We'd take turns buying thick slices of bread or Danish, depending on our moods.

Only two blocks to go—we were almost home. But how could we forget the ice-cream man, ringing his bell and inviting us to eat chocolate pops and sundaes made with nuts and fudge?

We'd make our selection depending on how much money we had left. (The sundaes were the most expensive.) Eating our ice cream, we'd wave goodbye, each of us walking up our different brownstone steps, each of us ready to face a mother who could never understand why we took so long to come home on Friday afternoons—and why we never ate our dinner that night with gusto.

What fertile ground for a food sensualist like me to grow!

"To your new life!"

—*The Daily Adele Dose*

• •

Date:

What I ate...for breakfast: _____
_____

What I ate...for my morning hard-chew snacks: _____
_____

What I ate...for lunch: _____
_____
_____

What I ate...for my afternoon soft chews: _____

What I ate...for dinner: _____
_____
_____

How I felt: _____
_____
_____

How I kept moving: _____
_____
_____

What I drank: _____
_____

Did I recognize a connection between my feelings and the
way I eat? _____

WEIGHTY ISSUES

Last week's weight: _____

Pounds lost: _____

New weight: _____

Don't forget those lost ounces and half pounds. They add up!

• •

Remember, the 5-Day Miracle Diet is a process. There is no on/off, start/stop, black/white. Remember to step back once in a while and view the process—and see how far you've come!

• •

A WEEK'S "POCKETFUL OF MIRACLES"

It's that time again! And the miracles keep coming. It's hard to believe that so many things can change in your life every week—and that nothing, not even the 5-Day Miracle Diet, ever stays the same.

You own your life—and you own your diet. Savor the moments when you act assertive, when you say no politely, when you add another ten sit-ups to your daily crunch.

Pick one special moment and write it down here. It will go far in helping you stay with my diet.

To help you think of another miracle, here's a quote from a client who has lost over sixty-five pounds:

• *This week I went into a regular store (a regular store!) to buy a dress for my sister's wedding. No one noticed me—and that was the best moment yet. Until, that is, I tried on a linen suit and came outside. People actually stared at me, and the salesperson told me I looked beautiful. Me!*

Now it's your turn: _____

_____

_____

"The 5-Day Miracle Diet is only words—until you decide to implement them!"

—*The Daily Adele Dose*

• •

Date:

What I ate...for breakfast: _____
_____
_____

What I ate...for my morning hard-chew snacks: _____
_____

What I ate...for lunch: _____
_____
_____
_____

What I ate...for my afternoon soft chews: _____

What I ate...for dinner: _____
_____
_____
_____

How I felt: _____
_____
_____

How I kept moving: _____
_____
_____

What I drank: _____
_____

Did I exercise when I woke up this morning? _____

Rosemary Lamb Chops

Most of the time, I recommend sticking to chicken and fish with veggies at mealtime. But every once in a while, you might see the image of a crisp, succulent lamb chop—and nothing less will do. This recipe is a fabulous take on the plain broiled lamb chop. It uses the aromatic flavorings of rosemary, shallots, and vinegar to create a tasty zing with every bite.

Enjoy these chops with a baked potato, a large green salad with one of my dressings, and a side dish such as Endive Étoile (page 70) or steamed yellow squash.

What you'll need:
- 1 tablespoon chopped garlic
- 1 tablespoon chopped rosemary
- 1 tablespoon chopped shallots
- 1 tablespoon balsamic vinegar
- 1 tablespoon chopped parsley
- 1 tablespoon chopped onion
- Salt and pepper to taste
- 1 tablespoon oil, preferably canola or olive
- 12 rib lamb chops (1 ounce each)

What you'll do:

Mix all the ingredients, except the oil and chops, in a large, nonreactive roasting pan. Add the lamb chops, cover, and marinate in the refrigerator for 6 hours.

Heat a large skillet until a drop of water sizzles in its center, add the oil and the lamb chops, and sauté the chops for 2 minutes on each side for rare meat, 3 minutes for medium-rare meat, and 4 minutes for well-done meat.

Serves 4 (3 chops each) for lunch or dinner. Men: Add 1 ounce low-fat sliced cheese to your salad.

"Emotional hunger, like boredom, rejection, frustration, and loneliness, needs an emotional food. Not popcorn, but a movie. Not chocolate, but a hot bath. Not a bagel, but a great big cuddle from your dog!"

—*The Daily Adele Dose*

• •

Date:

What I ate...for breakfast: _____

_____

_____

What I ate...for my morning hard-chew snacks: _____

_____

What I ate...for lunch: _____

_____

_____

_____

What I ate...for my afternoon soft chews: _____

What I ate...for dinner: _____

_____

_____

_____

How I felt: _____

_____

_____

How I kept moving: _____

_____

_____

What I drank: _____

_____

Did I feed my emotional hunger appropriately? _____

"I wasn't perfect. I was just fine!"

—A twenty-nine-year-old client
who's finally learned how to own the
5-Day Miracle Diet—and enjoy life!

Breathe In, Breathe Out

Sometimes the best ways to determine if you're making progress are the simplest. Forget scales, tape measures, clothes, and mirrors. Instead, walk up a flight of stairs. That's right. A flight of stairs. How do you feel? Are you out of breath? Or can you keep going? Feeling fit is a great way to know you're losing weight and getting healthy. All it takes is the "stairs test" to give you that extra "push-up" of motivation.

"Yes, you're getting the rhythm. Your feet feel lighter. And you're walking past your favorite food haunts without a thought. You must have completed five more days on the 5-Day Miracle Diet!"

—*The Daily Adele Dose*

* *

Date:

What I ate...for breakfast: _____

_____

_____

What I ate...for my morning hard-chew snacks: _____

_____

What I ate...for lunch: _____

_____

_____

_____

What I ate...for my afternoon soft chews: _____

What I ate...for dinner: _____

_____

_____

_____

How I felt: _____

_____

_____

How I kept moving: _____

_____

_____

What I drank: _____

_____

Did I pass up an early-morning muffin today? _____

BURN THOSE CALORIES AT WORK

Whoever said you can't lose weight at the office? Check this list and see if you've done any of the activities recently. Each one burns energy, takes muscle, and trims the mind:

- Walking to the bathroom, to the water cooler, to your office
- Running at the mouth at the board meeting
- Dancing a two-step in your boss's office
- Pulling your weight at the sales conference
- Passing the buck to your colleague
- Bending over backward to please your superiors
- Pushing for the bottom line
- Jumping to conclusions about the closed-door policy
- Hitting the nail on the head about the latest gossip
- Throwing your weight around at your subordinates

> *"Remember how incredible you felt when you had just finished your first five days?"*
>
> —*The Daily Adele Dose*

• •

Date:

What I ate...for breakfast: _____

_____

_____

What I ate...for my morning hard-chew snacks: _____

_____

What I ate...for lunch: _____

_____

_____

_____

What I ate...for my afternoon soft chews: _____

What I ate...for dinner: _____

_____

_____

_____

How I felt: _____

_____

_____

How I kept moving: _____

_____

_____

What I drank: _____

_____

Did I eat more vegetables than protein at lunch? _____

TEST YOUR PERSONAL GROWTH SAVVY

No, I'm not talking inches here (although pounds do enter the equation!). I'm talking about your inner self, your personal belief system, and how well you nurture and master your weaknesses. The 5-Day Miracle Diet is not a spiritual guide, but it can bring a serenity to your life. Because you learn to take care of yourself, to be selfish instead of self-less, you gain control over many aspects of your life—including, of course, the foods you eat. The result? Boundless energy, inner peace, and, of course, a lighter load with which to walk down the road each day.

Take a few minutes and see if your inner guide is talking true. See if your personal growth savvy is on the mark:

1. **You're working at your desk late at night. Everyone else has gone home. The cleaners are vacuuming in the distance. Your stomach is growling and you are feeling pretty sorry for yourself. You:**
(a) Call up a twenty-four-hour take-out place and order up some lo mein, an egg roll, fried rice—and a liter of Coke.
(b) Go out into the dark, look for food in the fridge, in someone's desk, in a cabinet—all the while reading other people's mail and generally being nosy.
(c) Take out your plastic bags of carrots and green beans and chomp away! You're almost done.

Your inner child might say go for the Chinese, but the adult who nurtures most definitely opts for (c), the bags of vegetables. Work is work, but it will soon be over.

2. **You're at home, looking for the misplaced phone number of the person you met last night. Riffling through your drawers, you find a chocolate bar. You:**
(a) Toss it in the garbage along with the outdated window cleaner ad.
(b) Grab it, rip it open, and chew! Who needs a date anyhow? You can live alone just fine!
(c) Frown, wondering how it got in the drawer. Feeling a *fathead* temptation, you stop looking for the phone number and decide to take the dog out for a walk. You'll find the number later.

The correct answer is (c), because you've recognized your frustration and your subsequent temptation, and instead of succumbing to a "Food tantrum," you've nurtured yourself in a healthy way. (a) is also acceptable. Although not a conscious decision, it still gets you to the same place!

"Sometimes you have to say goodbye to certain friends because they're toxic—like sugar!"

—*The Daily Adele Dose*

• •

Date:

What I ate...for breakfast: _____
_____
_____

What I ate...for my morning hard-chew snacks: _____
_____

What I ate...for lunch: _____
_____
_____
_____

What I ate...for my afternoon soft chews: _____

What I ate...for dinner: _____
_____
_____
_____

How I felt: _____
_____
_____

How I kept moving: _____
_____
_____

What I drank: _____
_____

*Did I time my hard chews correctly today?*_____

VEGETABLES FESTIVA

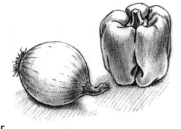

When I prepare this beautiful vegetable dish, I cannot help but think of celebrating. It's truly a festival of color, texture, taste, and spice. Enjoy this as a side dish to accompany Rosemary Lamb Chops (page 78), Chicken Oregon (page 254), or any of my other entrées. Add a salad with Tricolore Dressing (page 36), couscous, and a glass of sparkling water and you have a lunch or dinner fit for any occasion!

What you'll need:
- 1 cup broccoli florets
- 1 cup cauliflower florets
- ½ cup halved snow peas
- ½ cup halved green beans
- ½ cup julienne-cut red bell pepper
- 1 tablespoon extra-virgin olive oil
- 2 tablespoons chopped onions
- 1 tablespoon chopped garlic
- 1 tablespoon chopped rosemary
- 1 tablespoon chopped chives
- 2 tablespoons fines herbes

What you'll do:

Steam all the vegetables except the onions for 2 minutes. Set aside.

Heat the oil in a large nonstick skillet. Add the onions, garlic, and steamed vegetables and sauté for 2 minutes over medium heat. Add the rosemary, chives, and fines herbes and simmer for 5 minutes, stirring constantly.

Serves 4. Don't forget to add the oil toward your daily fat allotment.

MIRACLE DIET CHEF'S HINT: Fines herbes is a magnificent French blend of four herbs: dried parsley, chives, tarragon, and chervil. It adds an unusual flair to any dish, including Vegetables Festiva. You can purchase fines herbes in a specialty store or in your supermarket.

"My body, myself, my soul: I am what I feel!"

—*The Daily Adele Dose*

● ●

Date:

What I ate...for breakfast: _____

_____

What I ate...for my morning hard-chew snacks: _____

_____

What I ate...for lunch: _____

_____

_____

_____

What I ate...for my afternoon soft chews: _____

What I ate...for dinner: _____

_____

_____

_____

How I felt: _____

_____

_____

How I kept moving: _____

_____

_____

What I drank: _____

_____

Is my body image changing? _____

THE 5-DAY MIRACLE DIET'S
DECLARATION OF RIGHTS

I declare that I have control over my own life. I have the right to:

- Eat what I choose at the right times
- Send food back if it isn't what I ordered
- Politely and kindly refuse food that I do not want to eat
- Say no

TOO MUCH OF A GOOD THING

The best use for leftover "Foods You Adore" is to have none. Give them away. They're just too tempting—and you don't want them around when you're "coming back" but still in low blood sugar!

"I don't care if you don't think you lost enough weight in a given week. Weight loss is weight loss— and it adds up!"

—*The Daily Adele Dose*

• •

Date:

What I ate...for breakfast: _____
_____
_____

What I ate...for my morning hard-chew snacks: _____
_____

What I ate...for lunch: _____
_____
_____
_____

What I ate...for my afternoon soft chews: _____

What I ate...for dinner:_____
_____
_____
_____

How I felt: _____
_____
_____

How I kept moving: _____
_____
_____

What I drank: _____
_____

Did I weigh myself at the same time in the same clothes? _____

WEEKLY ASSESSMENT

WEIGHTY ISSUES

Last week's weight: _____

Pounds lost: _____

New weight: _____

Don't forget those lost ounces and half pounds. They add up!

• •

Remember that to live a good, exciting life, you must never stop learning—about people, about the world around you, and about food. Yes, food. You can always learn to eat better, smarter, and healthier throughout your life.

• •

A WEEK'S "POCKETFUL OF MIRACLES"

You know the expression. "When the going gets tough, the tough get going." I'm not quite sure what that means. I get this vision of a bunch of football players dropping the ball and running off the field.

I'd rather change it to "When the going gets tough, the tough *keep* going." And that's my point this week: sticking to it. Be mindless. Be a robot. Don't think about it. Keep your eating times straight. Eat your hard chews religiously. Eventually, you'll feel better. The bad cycle will end and the *fathead*'s army will retreat. And you'll have stayed on your diet, feeling even better than you did before!

That alone is miracle enough, but here's another example, from a West Coast reader:

• *There I was, crying my eyes out because my relationship broke up, but I didn't eat. Unbelievable. There's hope for me yet.*

Now it's your turn: _____

_____

_____

"Choice will defeat the fathead every time!"

—*The Daily Adele Dose*

• •

Date: _____

What I ate...for breakfast: _____
_____
_____

What I ate...for my morning hard-chew snacks: _____
_____

What I ate...for lunch: _____
_____
_____
_____

What I ate...for my afternoon soft chews: _____

What I ate...for dinner: _____
_____
_____
_____

How I felt: _____
_____
_____

How I kept moving: _____
_____
_____

What I drank: _____
_____

Did I actually feel the physiological feeling of hunger today? _____

TEST YOUR WEDDING SAVVY

You can't wait. Your best friend is getting married and you are so happy for her! You want to experience it all: crying at the service, drinking during the cocktail party, eating all the food, and dancing the night away. And, of course, you want to look absolutely smashing while all this activity is going on.

Well, there's no reason for you not to look smashing at your best friend's wedding. Especially if you've been on the 5-Day Miracle Diet. But there is life after the wedding. Believe it or not, you can have a fabulous time without getting into a blood-sugar hole. Let's see if you know some of my wedding tricks:

1. You walk into the dining room and discover that the first course is already sitting at your plate: strawberries and champagne. You:

(a) Take the strawberries out of the glass and put them on your butter dish to nibble later. You discreetly push the champagne away.

(b) Immediately guzzle the champagne and ask, "Does the glass next to you belong to anyone?"

(c) Decide there are too many other wonderful "Extras" at the party and you simply leave the first course, waiting for it to be whisked away.

This is a trick question. The correct answer is both (a) and (c), because either answer shows you made a choice and made the diet your own.

2. The gorgeous mocha-and-chocolate cake has been cut, and the waiters are bringing scrumptious slices around to everyone in the room. You:

(a) Can't wait because you've made the choice to eat the wedding cake as a "Food You Adore."

(b) Can't wait because you've already stuffed your face on the hors d'oeuvres, the bread basket, and the whiskey sours.

(c) Can't wait because it will mean the music will start again and you can get up to dance. After all, you've opted for your "Extra" to be the champagne, and you don't want to be tempted to eat more than the one "Food You Adore."

The correct answer is (a). It's appropriate and shows you have a handle on what you are doing. Although (c) sounds good in theory, there's a white-knuckled quality about it. So what if you eat more "Extras," this night? How often does your best friend get married!

"I don't allow the words good and bad. Just because you ate a cookie? If you killed someone that would be a different story. And it doesn't have a thing to do with food! A cookie?"

—*The Daily Adele Dose*

● ●

Date:

What I ate...for breakfast: _____

_____

_____

What I ate...for my morning hard-chew snacks: _____

_____

What I ate...for lunch: _____

_____

_____

_____

What I ate...for my afternoon soft chews: _____

What I ate...for dinner: _____

_____

_____

_____

How I felt: _____

_____

_____

How I kept moving: _____

_____

_____

What I drank: _____

_____

Did I write down my weekly "Pocketful of Miracles"? _____

STRETCH YOUR BODY AND YOUR SOUL

Try to perform my fifteen-minute stretch every day. You can do it in the morning to stay refreshed all day or in the evening to restore your inner balance. The more you do my stretch, the better you'll feel—and the more toned you'll become.

To make the fifteen-minute stretch (which is described in detail in *The 5-Day Miracle Diet*) a wonderful experience:

- Put on some light jazz or New Age music.
- Dim the lights in the room.
- Wear comfortable clothing.
- Keep your feet warm with sports socks, ballet slippers, or peds.
- Turn off your phone and keep the answering machine on low (so you won't be interrupted).
- Make sure you have enough space to move around!

Remember, this time is for *you*. Enjoy it and respect it!

• •

Living your life in good blood sugar means living your life to the fullest. It means having the ability to do more, feel more, and enjoy more. Isn't it worth sticking to the 5-Day Miracle Diet?

• •

"What are you waiting for?"

—*The Daily Adele Dose*

• •

Date:

What I ate...for breakfast: _____
_____
_____

What I ate...for my morning hard-chew snacks: _____
_____

What I ate...for lunch: _____
_____
_____
_____

What I ate...for my afternoon soft chews: _____

What I ate...for dinner: _____
_____
_____
_____

How I felt: _____
_____
_____

How I kept moving: _____
_____
_____

What I drank: _____
_____

Did I try Adele's fifteen-minute stretch? _____

Four-Mushroom Salad

The best part of the 5-Day Miracle Diet is the wonderful veggies you can eat to your heart's content (as long as you get those hard chews in)! This particular salad uses four robust mushrooms to create its flavor, 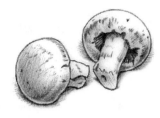 and there's not a drop of oil in sight. Enjoy the exotic textures and tastes of this salad with one of my chicken entrées or with my Twenty-Vegetable Soup for a light vegetarian repast.

What you'll need:
 1 cup low-fat chicken broth
 ½ cup balsamic vinegar
 ¼ cup white vinegar
 1 sliced garlic clove
 1 cup sliced shiitaki mushroom caps
 1 cup sliced white mushroom caps
 1 cup sliced portobello mushroom caps
 1 cup sliced cremini mushroom caps
    Salt and pepper to taste
 3 cups spinach leaves, washed, stemmed, and sliced

What you'll do:
 Bring the chicken broth, balsamic vinegar, white vinegar, and garlic to a boil in an 8-quart saucepan. Add all the mushrooms and simmer for 5 minutes. Add salt and pepper to taste.
 Remove from the heat and place in a bowl. Cover with plastic wrap and refrigerate for 6 hours.
 After 6 hours, taste the mixture. If it is not vinegary enough for your taste, add more balsamic vinegar.
 Spread the spinach leaves equally on four flat plates. Place the mushrooms over the spinach. Add some juice from the marinade to taste.

Serves 4.

"There is no such thing as a diet plateau. If you continue to stay with the basics of the 5-Day Miracle Diet, you might experience the occasional fluctuation, but plateaus will become a thing of the past!"

—*The Daily Adele Dose*

• •

Date:

What I ate...for breakfast: _____
_____
_____

What I ate...for my morning hard-chew snacks: _____
_____

What I ate...for lunch: _____
_____
_____
_____

What I ate...for my afternoon soft chews: _____

What I ate...for dinner:_____
_____
_____
_____

How I felt: _____
_____
_____

How I kept moving: _____
_____
_____

What I drank: _____
_____

Did I try switching to a different brand of water for variety?

_____

MANGIA! MANGIA!

Italian restaurants are perfectly fine places to go when you are on the 5-Day Miracle Diet. Really. You just have to know what to order—and what to stay clear of—for good blood-sugar control.

✔ Avoid anything with the word *Parmigiana* in it. That means lots of cheese and figuratively means fat, fat, fat. Ditto *scampi*. It means the dish will be doused in oil.

✔ If you are not stripping the carbs and it's an alternate night, ask for a side order of pasta with plain marinara sauce. (It's much smaller than the entrée size and will be less tempting!) Add one tablespoon of Parmesan cheese, a large salad tossed with balsamic vinegar, and a grilled chicken breast or shrimp dish, and you have a feast that feels like a Roman holiday.

✔ Order anything that's grilled: fish, chicken, veal, or lamb chops.

✔ Always ask what's in the sauce before you decide on a particular dish. Then you decide if you want to take a "dip": Order the dish with the sauce, but be prepared to either brush off the excess sauce or send it back. And you can always play it safe by asking the waiter to serve the sauce on the side. This "Sauce Dance" works best in a restaurant you know and trust!

✔ Many Italian restaurants today offer grilled vegetables as an appetizer. Order it as your main course, along with a shrimp cocktail and a salad (topped with balsamic vinegar). Add a chunk of plain Italian bread and you have a delicious meal (at much lower cost!).

✔ Try some San Pellegrino with lemon instead of white wine. It's sparkling and delicious. And it's water, so it's good for you, too.

Remember, you could always choose this night to have a **mangia, mangia** *"Extra":*

✔ Warm garlic bread
✔ Scampi
✔ A pasta dish with a fabulous sauce
✔ Stuffed mushrooms
✔ A glass of superb chianti

One word of advice: Keep it as light as possible. Your body will thank you tomorrow!

> *"Phrases like 'I don't deserve this,'...'I'm a horrible person,'...'I hate myself' don't belong in your vocabulary! Tear them up, stomp on them, and get aboard the 5-Day Miracle Diet plan!"*
>
> —*The Daily Adele Dose*

• •

Date:

What I ate...for breakfast: _____

_____

_____

What I ate...for my morning hard-chew snacks: _____

_____

What I ate...for lunch: _____

_____

_____

_____

What I ate...for my afternoon soft chews: _____

What I ate...for dinner: _____

_____

_____

_____

How I felt: _____

_____

_____

How I kept moving: _____

_____

_____

What I drank: _____

_____

Was I nice to myself today? _____

YOU LOOK GOOD, YOU FEEL GOOD, DAHLING!

When Billy Crystal played his nightclub lizard role on *Saturday Night Live*, he was only kidding. But the truth is that when you look good, you *do* feel good. And it has a cumulative effect.

If you feel well groomed and well dressed, you'll feel a solid sense of self. This, in turn, will strengthen your resolve on the 5-Day Miracle Diet.

And the more you are on my diet, the better you'll look and feel. Your cheeks will glow. Your eyes will sparkle. Your skin will be smoother. It's a win-win situation.

While you're waiting for those pounds to come off, here are some ways to look fabulous, dahling, fabulous:

✔ Wear clothes that fit! There's nothing worse than trying to wear something that's a tad too tight. Maybe no one else will notice, but it will have a devastating effect on you!

✔ Think monochromatic. If you're a woman, try one-color creations, from your blouse or sweater down to your stockings and shoes. It will make you look leaner and taller, too.

✔ Men should invest in a well-made, single-breasted suit, either a subtle pinstripe or a dark wool or linen. The buttons on the jacket should close easily, and there should be ample space under the arms.

✔ Leggings are today's answer for women. Just add a shirt that falls *below* your buttocks and you'll look ten pounds thinner. Promise!

✔ If you are a man, invest in a pair of well-fitting khaki chinos. They are like leggings. They'll move with you. They go with any color. They can be worn in any weather. And they don't have the "memory" of blue jeans (which will eventually sag in the wrong places and make you look as if you've gained weight!).

✔ Avoid horizontal stripes. They'll make any man or woman wider than he or she'd like!

✔ Black is not necessarily the only color choice for the overweight. Dark colors are flattering, true, but you can even get away with bright white if it's a well-fitting piece of clothing in a good material with classic lines.

✔ Accessorize, accessorize, accessorize. Women think up: pins, necklaces, and scarves strategically placed will keep eyes up—and away from hips and thighs. Men, too, can think up: with a classy but colorful tie.

✔ Alter a few of your favorite outfits. As people lose weight, many of them forget to alter their clothes. The result is baggy dresses and pants—which make them look just as heavy as before!

"Once your body is in good blood sugar, you can look at the 'real you' without fear, without revulsion, without the negative self-talk that stems from your body's bad-blood-sugar balance!"

—*The Daily Adele Dose*

• •

Date:

What I ate...for breakfast: _____
_____
_____

What I ate...for my morning hard-chew snacks: _____
_____

What I ate...for lunch: _____
_____
_____
_____

What I ate...for my afternoon soft chews: _____

What I ate...for dinner: _____
_____
_____
_____

How I felt: _____
_____
_____

How I kept moving: _____
_____
_____

What I drank: _____
_____

Did I try on a bathing suit today without making a face? _____

ICE CREAM BREAKER

I'd always known that the love of food was universal, but it took a trip to Germany with my husband to visually prove that food is a shared language all its own.

It was about ten years ago and Arthur, my husband, had to attend a business conference in Hanover. I decided to join him, not realizing how unspeakably boring some business conferences can be—especially when you don't understand the language!

One afternoon around three o'clock, I excused myself. I told Arthur I'd meet him back at the hotel at five, and while he conducted his business, I went out for a walk. I explored the town, browsing in flower shops and antique shops, smiling at the people on the street.

After about an hour, I looked at my watch. It was four, time for a soft chew to keep my blood sugar going until dinner. I stopped at a Novotel concession and ordered a bowl of strawberries.

In Germany, some of the restaurants are set up with long communal tables. You sit with other people, strangers, at the same table. I sat down, watching the people eating food with varying degrees of fat while I nibbled my berries. I glanced at my watch. It was the low-blood-sugar "magic" hour, when people get into a slump and need a nap or a sugar "hit." No wonder so many people in the restaurant were filling up on pastries and pie!

As my eyes roamed to the door, several distinguished-looking business people came into the restaurant. They were all well dressed, carrying attaché cases and looking very important. They didn't seem to know one another; they all simply sat down at my table because it was the emptiest one. I continued to eat my strawberries as each one, in turn, instructed the waiter in what seemed to be a serious tone.

A few minutes later, the waiter came out with an incredibly luscious-looking chocolate ice-cream confection. He set it down in front of one of the businessmen. Suddenly, the table became animated, cheerful. These strangers were all talking at once, laughing and pointing at the dessert, all of them acting like excited little kids. I still didn't know what they were saying, but by their gestures and their grins, it was obvious that they were talking about the businessman's dessert. They seemed to be congratulating him!

Sweets, that sugar "hit" in the middle of the afternoon, brought them together. The plain, ordinary restaurant had become a cabaret. I continued to eat my strawberries, marveling at the power of food!

Has anyone thought of bringing falafel and matzo ball soup to the Middle East talks and serving them as a late-afternoon snack?

"There's only one way to fight the 'blahs' and the 'need to feed' symptoms of bad blood sugar. Get in great blood sugar—with the 5-Day Miracle Diet!"

—*The Daily Adele Dose*

• •

Date:

What I ate...for breakfast: _____

_____

What I ate...for my morning hard-chew snacks: _____

_____

What I ate...for lunch: _____

_____

_____

What I ate...for my afternoon soft chews: _____

What I ate...for dinner: _____

_____

_____

How I felt: _____

_____

_____

How I kept moving: _____

_____

What I drank: _____

_____

Did I go through the day without a single craving? _____

WEEKLY ASSESSMENT

WEIGHTY ISSUES

Last week's weight: _____

Pounds lost: _____

New weight: _____

*Don't forget those lost ounces and half
pounds. They add up!*

● ●

*Who thought up the size of a dinner plate? Not me, not you.
Just because your entrée fills the surface doesn't mean
it eventually has to fill your stomach. Leave some food on your
plate. It will make you feel powerful: you have
control of your food!*

● ●

A WEEK'S "POCKETFUL OF MIRACLES"

*N*o! Another week already? Look back at the week just past. Do you
think you had more hits than misses? Was it a good week? A fair week?
Or a week where the *fathead* kept trying to trap you?

Analyze, analyze, analyze. Even if you had one or two *fathead*
encounters, there's always triumph in the midst of despair. Just the fact
that here you are, ready to begin a new week, is a triumph—and a
miracle in its own right!

Whatever the week that was, think of just one important "miracle"
that was a catalyst to keep you on the right path.

Here's one a client told me last week:

• *My girlfriend had just broken up with me. I could have walked into a corner bar and drunk enough to stumble home—or I could have gone to the
gym. I picked the latter, and boy that Lifecycle was sorry! (But I wasn't!)*

Now it's your turn: _____

_____

_____

"If you accurately follow my stripping the carbs program for three to five days, you will no longer crave that pasta with so much passion. I am sure of it!"

—*The Daily Adele Dose*

• •

Date:

What I ate...for breakfast: _____

_____

_____

What I ate...for my morning hard-chew snacks: _____

_____

What I ate...for lunch: _____

_____

_____

_____

What I ate...for my afternoon soft chews: _____

What I ate...for dinner: _____

_____

_____

_____

How I felt: _____

_____

_____

How I kept moving: _____

_____

_____

What I drank: _____

_____

Did I eat pasta on an alternate day—or on a once-a-week basis if I'm a "carbohydrate addict"? _____

NAPA VALLEY CHICKEN

I call this my "California-style" chicken because it combines different textures and foods to create a new taste sensation. It's also a little-known fact that walnuts love to grow in the valleys that nurture the vineyards. The small amount of chopped walnuts here adds a nutty, crunchy flavor to the dish without sacrificing the low-fat or low-caloric value.

It's a lovely and different dish to serve to company with a baked sweet potato and one of my new side dishes, such as Vegetables Festiva (page 86).

What you'll need:
   4   tablespoons extra-virgin olive oil
   8   sliced scallions
  16   sliced shiitaki mushroom caps
  ¼   cup chopped walnuts
  24   ounces skinless, boneless chicken breast
   4   ripe plum (Roma) tomatoes, sliced in sections
       Salt and pepper to taste
  ¾   cup low-fat chicken broth

What you'll do:

Heat 2 tablespoons of the olive oil in a nonstick skillet and sauté the scallions, shiitaki caps, and walnuts over medium heat for 3 minutes. Remove from the pan and set aside.

Using the same skillet, add the remaining 2 tablespoons of oil and the chicken breasts. Sauté the chicken over medium heat until brown on both sides.

Add the tomatoes, salt, and pepper, then the scallion mixture, and then the chicken broth. Bring to a boil.

Serves 4 (male-sized portions). Women: Slice off about 2 ounces chicken and set aside. Wrap in foil and eat for breakfast or add to lunch or dinner the next day.

"The confidence you find on the 5-Day Miracle Diet can be quite a turn-on to a spouse or lover!"

—*The Daily Adele Dose*

• •

Date:

What I ate...for breakfast: _____
_____
_____

What I ate...for my morning hard-chew snacks: _____
_____

What I ate...for lunch: _____
_____
_____
_____

What I ate...for my afternoon soft chews: _____

What I ate...for dinner: _____
_____
_____
_____

How I felt: _____
_____
_____

How I kept moving: _____
_____
_____

What I drank: _____
_____

Did I try an exotic starch today? _____

SOUTH OF THE BORDER

You don't have to steer clear of Mexican restaurants when you're on the 5-Day Miracle Diet. The sangría and the margaritas might make your blood sugar have a nervous breakdown, but there are dishes that, believe it or not, will keep your blood sugar balanced—while you have a great time with your friends or family!

Get away as fast as a Mexican jumping bean from:

✔ Refried beans. They're cooked with lard . . . twice!
✔ Nachos and tortilla chips. As with those ubiquitous Chinese noodles, have the waiter take them away—or keep them out of arm's reach.
✔ And don't even bother to memorize the name chimichangas. They're deep-fried burritos!

Build up your appetite with a Mexican hat dance for:

✔ Salsa . . . and more salsa
✔ Onion, avocado, and tomato salad with dressing on the side
✔ Seviche, which is spicy, marinated fish
✔ Any kind of chicken dish with *poblano* or *serrano* in its name (the chicken will be roasted with herbs, tomatoes, and hot spices). Ask the waiter to hold the cheese.
✔ Steamed rice
✔ And you can even order a chicken or beef taco. Simply eat the inside and leave the highly glycemic (and soggy) taco shell behind.

Or let your soul soar to the magical guitars and delicious "Extras," such as:

✔ A frozen margarita (and keep it to one!)
✔ Super-hot nachos (as an appetizer used as an entrée)
✔ Beef or chicken tortilla platter (complete with rice and beans)
✔ Sausage and cheese casserole (but don't eat all of it!)
✔ Guacamole-and-sour-cream dip (as much as is necessary to keep you happy)

*"**There is no such thing as a relapse!***"*

—*The Daily Adele Dose*

• •

Date:

What I ate...for breakfast: _____
_____
_____

What I ate...for my morning hard-chew snacks: _____
_____

What I ate...for lunch: _____
_____
_____
_____

What I ate...for my afternoon soft chews: _____

What I ate...for dinner: _____
_____
_____
_____

How I felt: _____
_____
_____

How I kept moving: _____
_____
_____

What I drank: _____
_____

Did I bring my water and hard chews on the plane? _____

NO: A LITTLE WORD WITH A BIG MEANING

Charlotte's story is a common one, especially among women. On the surface, she seemed to be doing just fine. She'd been on the 5-Day Miracle Diet for about six weeks and had lost ten pounds.

But more important than the weight was Charlotte's attitude: She had changed from a shy, quiet secretary into a poised, confident woman.

Anyone who saw her or talked to her would know that Charlotte was making progress. She knew the diet plan by heart; she had no cravings when she stuck to the rules of the 5-Day Miracle Diet.

But something was wrong. Charlotte couldn't get past these ten pounds. Six *more* weeks went by and she still weighed the same. She'd "forget" a hard chew one afternoon. She'd sneak a frozen yogurt after dinner. Charlotte didn't gain—but she didn't lose, either. She was frustrated; she felt like a failure. "What's wrong with me?" she asked.

Both of us knew the answer: the *fathead*. Charlotte's psychological issues were all about her need to please. In fact, she found it almost impossible to say no when someone asked her to do something—even when it was bad for her mental health. She couldn't bear the disapproval, the disappointment she might inflict. In other words, Charlotte's whole sense of self was completely dependent on others. She needed reassurance constantly. "You like me! You really like me!" was her deepest wish.

Unfortunately, after the yes came the inner rage, which she literally swallowed with a sesame bagel, a "tiny" chocolate chip cookie, and other dollops of not-so-sweet self-sabotage.

It was a vicious cycle. The more Charlotte said yes, the more she ate her rage. "*Chomp!* I hate being at the mercy of others. *Chew!* Why can't I say no for once! *Swallow!* I have no pride. I am nothing."

Once Charlotte understood the dynamics of her **Need-to-Please fathead**, she was able to get beyond it. She tentatively and politely said no to a friend who wanted her to do an errand, to a boss who made an impossible demand—and learned that it didn't mean the end of the world.

It wasn't long before Charlotte was saying no to sweets and extra carbs, too. The rage was gone, and she no longer had to eat her feelings. Finally, *she* was in control. Finally, she was living her life, her way, and loving every moment!

"Are you ready to feel better than you ever have?"

—*The Daily Adele Dose*

• •

Date:

What I ate...for breakfast: _____
_____
_____

What I ate...for my morning hard-chew snacks: _____
_____

What I ate...for lunch: _____
_____
_____
_____

What I ate...for my afternoon soft chews: _____

What I ate...for dinner: _____
_____
_____
_____

How I felt: _____
_____
_____

How I kept moving: _____
_____
_____

What I drank: _____
_____

Was I more focused and more able to concentrate today? _____

Fava Bean Zing Dip

One of the best ways to ward off boredom is with a zingy new dip to add
zip to your carrots, string beans,
and cabbage—and I am always
on the lookout for interesting
new dipping sauces. This unusual
bean dip does the trick, without oil!

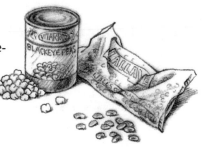

What you'll need:
- 1 cup canned fava beans, drained
- ½ cup canned white or red cannellini beans, strained
- 2 tablespoons balsamic vinegar
- 1 tablespoon fresh lemon juice
- 1 tablespoon chopped basil
    Pinch of oregano, fresh or dried
    Salt and pepper to taste

What you'll do:

Mix all the ingredients in a blender or food processor for 2 to 3 minutes. Pour into a small dish. Serve with fresh crudités.

Men: Use three-quarters of the dip as a starchy vegetable. Women: Use
half of the dip as a starchy vegetable. Save the remainder in the refrigerator to dip veggies into during the week.

"Never eat less than the basic 5-Day Miracle Diet. You want to stay strong, healthy, and in good blood sugar!"

—*The Daily Adele Dose*

• •

Date:

What I ate...for breakfast: _____

_____

_____

What I ate...for my morning hard-chew snacks: _____

_____

What I ate...for lunch: _____

_____

_____

_____

What I ate...for my afternoon soft chews: _____

What I ate...for dinner: _____

_____

_____

_____

How I felt: _____

_____

_____

How I kept moving: _____

_____

_____

What I drank: _____

_____

Did I say,"I'd love to, but not right now—I'm stuffed" to a friend who'd made me dinner? _____

Like a Big Pizza...Slice

The rumors are true. You can eat pizza on the 5-Day Miracle Diet. We all know pizza's high in fat, but so many people love it that I allow one slice, once a week, for lunch or dinner. After all, there are worse things. The mozzarella cheese helps "save" your blood sugar balance. And the crust is considered a starch. (Of course, make sure you count one slice as part of your daily allotment of protein and starch.) But any more than one slice per week and you're into "Extra" territory.

Always accompany your slice of pizza with a salad topped with balsamic vinegar or lemon as a dressing (to counteract the oily pizza). It will fill you up—not out—as you satisfy your pizza, pizza pleasure.

"White-knuckled motivation belongs in the boxing ring. Not here!"

—The Daily Adele Dose

• •

Date:

What I ate...for breakfast: _____

_____

_____

What I ate...for my morning hard-chew snacks: _____

_____

What I ate...for lunch: _____

_____

_____

_____

What I ate...for my afternoon soft chews: _____

What I ate...for dinner: _____

_____

_____

_____

How I felt: _____

_____

_____

How I kept moving: _____

_____

_____

What I drank: _____

_____

Did I analyze and figure out a strategy for an old fathead *issue of mine?*_____

FATTY THOUGHTS

These fatty thoughts are like fatty tissue. They keep you from losing weight—while they make you want to eat *more* ("Feed me, feed me" those fat cells say, just as the *fathead* does in your mind!).

Here are some fatty thoughts that will just keep you down. Do they sound familiar?

- Only three pounds! I have so much weight still to go.
- It's not fair. How come some people eat anything they want and never gain weight?
- I have too much weight to lose. Why bother?
- I've been on so many diets and they never worked. This one won't either.
- Why don't I just admit it? I'm big and fat and I always will be!

Yecch! The negative energy is enough to suck you into a black hole. But fatty thoughts can be turned into lean machines, positive counterpunches that keep the fathead *silent (while the 5-Day Miracle Diet takes care of the body). Here are some examples:*

- Three pounds isn't a lot, but it all adds up. It's a great start!
- So I'm not blessed with a super metabolism. I don't look like Cindy Crawford, either. Not many people do. But I'm healthy, I'm loved, and I have the 5-Day Miracle Diet to keep me revved up!
- Of course no diet worked for me. The food cravings were always crawling all over me! This time it's different. I'm just not tempted to eat the wrong things. This isn't a diet. It's a life!
- We think so little of ourselves sometimes—and it always hinges on weight. When did five or ten or fifteen pounds make us a better person? I don't need to be on a diet to feel good about myself. I have the 5-Day Miracle Diet—and it's changing the way my body, my heart, and my soul think about food. That's a good start for me!

"The fathead is only as strong as you let it be!"

—*The Daily Adele Dose*

• •

Date:

What I ate...for breakfast: _____
_____
_____

What I ate...for my morning hard-chew snacks: _____
_____

What I ate...for lunch: _____
_____
_____
_____

What I ate...for my afternoon soft chews: _____

What I ate...for dinner: _____
_____
_____
_____

How I felt: _____
_____
_____

How I kept moving: _____
_____
_____

What I drank: _____
_____

Did I do some deep-breathing exercises at my desk? _____

*I*t's hard to believe yet another month has flown by and the 5-Day Miracle Diet is still doing its magic! In fact, I'm sure that by now you have the diet-plan basics down to a science. You know how to eat: It's ingrained in your brain. But wait, why are some days just fine and others filled with craving braying? You've been following the diet perfectly. So what's going on?

Well, as you probably suspect, it's the *fathead* at work, those sometimes subtle sabotages we pull on ourselves because of unresolved issues from our past, unexpressed emotions, poor self-images, and stress-induced anxiety. And because you are now feeling terrific, you just might be facing these *fathead* issues for the very first time! Suddenly, you are facing your fears instead of hiding behind a bowl of pasta.

During this month, think of yourself as a knight in shining armor, facing the *fathead* dragon and determined to succeed. Take more time to fill in the "How I felt" section of your journal. Try to remember when a craving hit. What were you doing? Who were you with? What had occurred immediately before the need for food?

Asking yourself these questions will help you understand the dynamics behind that ubiquitous 25 percent of weight-loss mania called the *fathead*. And use the strategies and tools I suggest in *The 5-Day Miracle Diet*. They work!

Inch-by-Inch

Bust/chest: _____   Upper arms: _____

Wrists: _____   Waist: _____

Abdomen: _____   Hips and buttocks: _____

IN A WORD...

Sum up your monthly experience in one or two words. Use it as your "mantra" in the month to come. It's easy now that you've made the 5-Day Miracle Diet yours to keep! Here's one of my favorites:

At last. I am in charge of my own life!

What's your good word?

_____

Shout it out. You should feel proud!

Are you "losing it" instead of losing it? Stress can make you retain water—and it also makes you look at yourself with an overly critical eye. Get rid of the stress with a good workout, good blood sugar, a calming walk, or an enjoyable book, and you'll realize you've been losing "it" (the weight) all along!

It's said that faith can move mountains.

Faith in yourself can move "a mountain of bad self-image," regardless of your weight. In fact, once our self-image has changed, the weight becomes unimportant.

WEEKLY ASSESSMENT

WEIGHTY ISSUES

Last week's weight: _____

Pounds lost: _____

New weight: _____

Don't forget those lost ounces and half pounds. They add up!

• •

There's nothing like in-season fruits and vegetables. They are at their peak: fresh, succulent, and ripe. Exploit the seasons and the healthy foods they represent!

• •

A WEEK'S "POCKETFUL OF MIRACLES"

Miracles don't grow on trees. But apples do. And they're one of the best hard chews around. By now you know the importance of those hard chews on the 5-Day Miracle Diet. Eating your hard chews at the right times can make all the difference in your weight loss. If you don't eat them on time, you're looking at a craving ready to happen.

Because they are so important, I'd like to use this week's "miracle box" to reinforce your hard-chew habit. Maybe you went away on vacation and you managed to pack some plastic bags filled with string beans and apples. Or maybe you simply managed to eat your hard chews on time—for the first time on the diet plan! Whatever it is, look to the miracle and write it down. Here's one from a man who had the hardest time fitting in his hard-chew snacks:

• *I was late for a business lunch, so I grabbed a carrot from my desk and ran outside. And I didn't care who saw me chomping away!*

Now it's your turn: _____

_____

_____

"There's nothing like the feeling of well-being, the energy, and the vitality that come from living in good blood sugar—not to mention the delight as your weight drops off!"

—*The Daily Adele Dose*

● ●

Date:

What I ate...for breakfast: _____
_____
_____

What I ate...for my morning hard-chew snacks: _____
_____

What I ate...for lunch: _____
_____
_____
_____

What I ate...for my afternoon soft chews: _____

What I ate...for dinner: _____
_____
_____
_____

How I felt: _____
_____
_____

How I kept moving: _____
_____
_____

What I drank: _____
_____

Did I leave some of my protein and starch on my plate at the restaurant? _____

THERE'S GOING TO BE A PARTY—
AT YOUR HOUSE

It's the moment of truth: It's your turn to return the invitation. You have to cook a meal for all those friends who had you at their house (two or three times). You used to enjoy cooking, but that was back in the days when you used to use butter as a liberal condiment and everything was cooked in heavy cream, heavy oil, and heavy metal.

You could go out and buy a low-fat cookbook, but many of those recipes contain a lot of sugar to compensate for the absence of oil.

You could serve a platter of tofu and veggies, but that's hardly a memorable meal.

You could even forget all the good work you've done on the 5-Day Miracle Diet and make your special Chicken Kiev and pecan pie—and eat it all up before the guests even arrive.

I have a better idea: Why not go for some of the scrumptious recipes in this book? Red Snapper Crazy Water (page 144) or Chicken Oregon (page 254) is wonderful to serve to company. Simply double the recipe if it's dinner for six or eight. And remember to keep your portion within your daily allotment. Ditto the side dishes, such as Endive Étoile (page 70) or Asparagus Fromage (page 173). You can start the meal with crudités and a dip (which you don't have to eat) and some shrimp on ice.

And for dessert you can always choose a "Food You Adore." My favorite—and a real crowd pleaser, too: "The Devil Made Me Do It" Chocolate Cake. Just don't forget to give the leftovers to one of your friends to take home!

Serve some chilled wine and iced sparkling water with a slice of lemon...and you have a lovely meal, worthy of your guests, your home—and you! Enjoy.

"I've been around and I've learned a few important truths—including the fact that dieting has nothing to do with willpower! "

—*The Daily Adele Dose*

• •

Date:

What I ate...for breakfast: _____
_____
_____

What I ate...for my morning hard-chew snacks: _____
_____

What I ate...for lunch: _____
_____
_____
_____

What I ate...for my afternoon soft chews: _____

What I ate...for dinner: _____
_____
_____
_____

How I felt: _____
_____
_____

How I kept moving: _____
_____
_____

What I drank: _____
_____

Did I give myself a small nonfood reward item, like a CD or a wacky tie? _____

SUCK IN YOUR CHEEKS!

So maybe you haven't seen cheekbones on your face since you were ten years old. Maybe you never had them. It doesn't matter. You can still look pretty and well groomed, even if you don't go the Cher route. Here are some slimming face tips from the makeup experts:

✔ Stay away from short, round-styled hair; you'll look like a lollipop. Leave that to the group on *Friends*. Instead, opt for layers around your cheeks. A glamorous twist will add height and stature.

✔ Avoid bangs. You'll look like a chipmunk. Instead, have your hairdresser cut the hair around your face in long, loose layers.

✔ Concentrate on your eyes. Have your eyebrows professionally shaped and wear a neutral, light shadow to make your eyes "leap out." Add a smidgen of eyeliner and smudge-proof mascara and no one will ever get past your Bette Davis eyes.

✔ Keep your makeup simple. Pancake makeup in two-toned colors to create the "cheekbone effect" is passé. Simply use a foundation in your color range. Top with a neutral blusher and translucent powder.

✔ Special strokes for applying blusher are also out-of-date. Just blush wherever and whenever you want. (But make sure it's a subtle color. Too much red and you'll look like a clown!)

✔ Don't make the mistake of wearing a bright lipstick to compete with your eyes. Instead, wear a soft rose or beige color with a drop of gloss. Forget frosted lipsticks. They'd make even Isabella Rosellini look dowdy!

"The biggest high of all is when you decide to make a life change—and stay with the 5-Day Miracle Diet!"

—*The Daily Adele Dose*

• •

Date: _____

What I ate...for breakfast: _____
_____
_____

What I ate...for my morning hard-chew snacks: _____
_____

What I ate...for lunch: _____
_____
_____
_____

What I ate...for my afternoon soft chews: _____

What I ate...for dinner: _____
_____
_____
_____

How I felt: _____
_____
_____

How I kept moving: _____
_____
_____

What I drank: _____
_____

Did I recognize a new fathead *saboteur today—and stop it in its tracks?* _____

CAMICIA SALMON

A marvelous recipe with an unusual sauce.

What you'll need:

Salt and pepper to taste
1 (2-pound) Savoy cabbage
(It must be Savoy to provide delicious results!)
2 tablespoons extra-virgin olive oil
½ cup chopped onion
8 chopped basil leaves
1 tablespoon chopped thyme (or ½ tablespoon dried)

2 tablespoons chopped parsley
2 lightly beaten egg whites
1 tablespoon grated Parmesan or Romano cheese
4 (4-ounce) center-cut salmon steaks

For *Camicia* Sauce:

1 tablespoon extra-virgin olive oil
2 tablespoons chopped onion
2 chopped red bell peppers
3 chopped ripe plum (Roma) tomatoes

1 tablespoon chopped parsley
1 tablespoon chopped basil
Salt and pepper to taste

What you'll do:

Preheat the oven to 400°F. Fill an 8-quart saucepan with enough salted water to cover the cabbage and bring to a boil. Place the cabbage in the boiling, salted water. Remove 4 leaves after 5 minutes. Set aside. Boil the remaining cabbage until tender and pliable when pricked with a fork. Shred the cabbage. You'll need 2 cups. Set aside.

Heat the oil in a large skillet. Add the onions and shredded cabbage and sauté until soft, about 5 minutes. Remove pan from stove. Add the basil, thyme, parsley, egg whites, cheese, salt, and pepper and stir to combine.

Spread the set-aside leaves on a flat surface. Place a salmon steak in the center of each leaf. Sprinkle with salt and pepper. Cover the salmon steak with the cabbage mixture in the pan and wrap the leaf around the salmon/cabbage mixture. Bake for 10 minutes.

To make the sauce:

Heat a 4-quart saucepan over high heat until a drop of water sizzles in its center. Add the oil, onions, and peppers and sauté until the onions are golden. Add the tomatoes, parsley, and basil. Bring to a boil, then simmer for 5 minutes. Put the mixture in a blender or food processor and purée. Squeeze the juice out through a strainer. Add salt and pepper. Serve sauce underneath the cabbage leaf or on top.

Serves 4. Men: Add extra protein at lunch and dinner. And don't forget to add the oil toward your daily allotment of fat.

"A sweater is only as good as the raw materials used in making it—just like your 'basic' choices on the 5-Day Miracle Diet!"

—The Daily Adele Dose

• •

Date:

What I ate...for breakfast: _____
_____
_____

What I ate...for my morning hard-chew snacks: _____
_____

What I ate...for lunch: _____
_____
_____
_____

What I ate...for my afternoon soft chews: _____

What I ate...for dinner: _____
_____
_____
_____

How I felt: _____
_____
_____

How I kept moving: _____
_____
_____

What I drank: _____
_____

Did I put a Post-It on my door to remind me to take my hard chews to work? _____

GO FISH!

Tune your taste buds in to something different with a variety of fish. Sure, tuna, salmon, scallops, and red snapper are all delicious, but why not try one of these for a new taste sensation? (Yes, it's true. Not all fish tastes alike!)

- *Rainbow trout.* It has a light, flavorful taste.

- *Whitefish.* Tastes sweet!

- *Orange roughy.* Cute enough to eat, with its orange skin and mild taste.

- *Pompano.* Sometimes called the king of fish. The texture is creamy and the taste is somewhat sharp.

- *Shark.* No, not the Great White. Mako shark actually tastes like steak. Try it as a low-fat, low-calorie substitute on your barbecue kabobs.

- *Porgy.* This saltwater fish is firm and chewy. It's great on the grill.

- *Catfish.* A knockout sweet sensation, catfish is *the* fish in many popular restaurants. Try yours grilled with hot peppers or Tabasco sauce.

- *Bluefish.* This blue (!) fish, a staple in the islands off the coast of New England, is great in tomato-based sauces. Marinate for twenty-four hours in crushed tomato, chopped onions, and Italian seasonings before cooking. Lovely!

"The diet becomes yours not *when I tell you to do a list of things, but when you want to do them. That's the point when the diet becomes a part of your life for good!"*

—*The Daily Adele Dose*

• •

Date:

What I ate...for breakfast: _____
_____
_____

What I ate...for my morning hard-chew snacks: _____
_____

What I ate...for lunch: _____
_____
_____
_____

What I ate...for my afternoon soft chews: _____

What I ate...for dinner: _____
_____
_____
_____

How I felt: _____
_____
_____

How I kept moving: _____
_____
_____

What I drank: _____
_____

Did I try one of Adele's delicious recipes? _____

CHARLOTTE SALAD

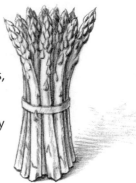

Over the years, the chefs at Restaurant Navona added a little of this and a little of that and came up with Charlotte Salad. I love its different textures, its intriguing combination of vegetables, and its graceful presentation. And it doesn't hurt that the dish—and its dressing—have the same name as my granddaughter!

An elegant, stylized salad. Serve it and impress company with (what else!) Charlotte Dressing! Enjoy.

What you'll need:
¼ cup chopped asparagus (keep twelve 3-inch tips intact)
 1 cup chopped endive (keep 12 large leaves intact)
 1 cup chopped arugula
½ cup chopped radicchio (keep 12 large leaves intact)
 6 chopped mushroom caps
¼ cup chopped roasted bell pepper or chopped pimientos
½ cup romaine
    Charlotte Dressing (page 132)

What you'll do:

Boil the asparagus, including the tips, for 3 minutes. Chill. Set tips aside.

Mix the chopped endive, arugula, radicchio, mushrooms, asparagus, and romaine in a large bowl.

Add Charlotte Dressing to the salad.

To serve:

Place some salad in the middle of each serving dish. Put roasted peppers or pimientos over the salad. Along the sides of the salad, arrange 1 radicchio leaf and 1 endive leaf. Place 3 asparagus tips inside each endive leaf. Serve—or rather, present!

Serves 4. Don't forget to add the salad dressing toward your daily allotment of fat.

"Choose as many vegetarian meals as you desire. I love to eat one once a day!"

—The Daily Adele Dose

• •

Date:

What I ate...for breakfast: _____
_____
_____

What I ate...for my morning hard-chew snacks: _____
_____

What I ate...for lunch: _____
_____
_____
_____

What I ate...for my afternoon soft chews: _____

What I ate...for dinner: _____
_____
_____
_____

How I felt: _____
_____
_____

How I kept moving: _____
_____
_____

What I drank: _____
_____

Did I make sure I mixed vegetables with vegetarian proteins, like low-fat soy cheese, tofu, or beans? _____

CHARLOTTE DRESSING

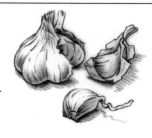

I love this Restaurant Navona dressing so much that I use it with almost everything. Drizzle it over fresh greens, tricolored salads, endive-and-arugula salads, or chicken breasts and fish for a delicious marinade—and especially on my Charlotte Salad, of course. (See page 128.)

What you'll need:
- ½ teaspoon balsamic vinegar
- 2 tablespoons extra-virgin olive oil
- 2 tablespoons red wine vinegar
- 1 tablespoon Dijon mustard
  Pinch of chopped garlic
  Pinch of finely chopped fresh oregano, or dried
  Salt and pepper to taste

What you'll do:
Mix all the ingredients in a bowl, using a whisk. Store in a covered container in the refrigerator. Shake before using.

Serves 4. Don't forget to add the dressing toward your daily fat allotment.

MIRACLE DIET CHEF'S HINT: Extra-virgin olive oil might cost a bit more, but it's worth it. "Extra-virgin" means that only the best hand-picked olives are used and that the process of making the oil itself is natural, or "cold-pressed" without any chemicals or heat. It has a robust flavor and offers the most taste.

> *"It's so exciting! Your body is going to change, and you—your personality and your mind—will grow the more you stay with my 5-Day Miracle Diet!"*
>
> *—The Daily Adele Dose*

• •

Date:

What I ate...for breakfast: _____

_____

_____

What I ate...for my morning hard-chew snacks: _____

_____

What I ate...for lunch: _____

_____

_____

_____

What I ate...for my afternoon soft chews: _____

What I ate...for dinner: _____

_____

_____

_____

How I felt: _____

_____

_____

How I kept moving: _____

_____

_____

What I drank: _____

_____

Did I try eating a chop instead of the pasta at the Italian restaurant? _____

WEIGHTY ISSUES

Last week's weight: _____

Pounds lost: _____

New weight: _____

Don't forget those lost ounces and half pounds. They add up!

• •

The next time you go out to eat with your friends or family, order first. You won't be tempted to order that fattening dish with the sauce your friend is having: You've already taken care of yourself in a positive way!

• •

A WEEK'S "POCKETFUL OF MIRACLES"

I remember the first few months of my experiences on the 5-Day Miracle Diet. I knew I was on the right track, that the foods I chose to eat, the times, and the combinations were balancing my blood chemistry, but I hadn't realized just how profound the impact of a balanced blood-sugar chemistry was. I knew it would make me feel good, but I felt better than good, better than great; I felt fabulous.

I had to share this discovery with others. While the scientist in me needed to prove my theories and put them into practice, the "child" in me wanted to run down the street to tell everyone the news.

Here's one of my earliest miracles, one I'll never forget:

• *I was driving home on the Long Island Expressway. It was late afternoon, the time I usually felt drowsy and needed to keep myself awake. Instead, I picked up my tape recorder and began making notes about my diet. I was so excited, I almost drove the car off the road!*

Now it's your turn: _____

_____

_____

"Toss out your bagels, your bananas, and your low-fat cookies. The 5-Day Miracle Diet will change your need for them—for good."

—The Daily Adele Dose

• •

Date:

What I ate...for breakfast: _____

_____

_____

What I ate...for my morning hard-chew snacks: _____

_____

What I ate...for lunch: _____

_____

_____

_____

What I ate...for my afternoon soft chews: _____

What I ate...for dinner: _____

_____

_____

_____

How I felt: _____

_____

_____

How I kept moving: _____

_____

_____

What I drank: _____

_____

Did I say no to a chocolate candy when it was offered? _____

SHOOT THE SHOULDS

Those *fatheads* are persistent creatures. You can be in the best blood sugar in the world and they'll still be around, waiting to pounce if you don't yet "own" the 5-Day Miracle Diet.

One of their best tricks is the *"Mighty Shoulds."* Personally, I believe that the word *should* should be sent into a room with *perfect, never,* and *I'll be back on Thursday to finish the job.* Let these absolutes fight over who's the most destructive among themselves.

The point is that nobody's perfect and we don't live in a perfect world.

Never is a long, long time—and it can be a pretty tight-fitting box.

Should is the guilty cousin of *could*—and it has no bearing on real life except when mothers want children to clean their rooms. Shoulds can set you up for diet failure.

Here are some shoulds that have been floating around the diet world a long, long time—along with the way the 5-Day Miracle Diet banishes them.

The Should Talk	The Adele Tell
I should exercise every single day.	I'll try to exercise at least once this week—or maybe just try to add some natural activities to my everyday routines.
I should forgo that fabulous-looking chocolate cake.	I think I'll eat this as my "Food You Adore"!
I should eat my salad with vinegar.	I love salad dressing. I'll just ask for it on the side and drizzle it on my greens.
I should eat fish because it's lower in calories. I should eat it dry.	I think I'll try the grilled chicken breast with veggies. I'll wipe off any excess sauce.
I should stay home so I won't eat any fattening foods.	I'll concentrate on dancing at the party. And I'll make sure it's a "Food You Adore" night. Maybe I'll even make my dinner a platter of hors d'oeuvres.

"I can tell you five hundred things to do to help you get in good blood sugar, but if I tell you them all at once, or even spaced out over a couple of weeks, you'll give up. I'd rather give you ten good hints to keep you going—and you will keep going!"

—*The Daily Adele Dose*

• •

Date:

What I ate...for breakfast: _____
_____
_____

What I ate...for my morning hard-chew snacks: _____
_____

What I ate...for lunch: _____
_____
_____
_____

What I ate...for my afternoon soft chews: _____

What I ate...for dinner: _____
_____
_____
_____

How I felt: _____
_____
_____

How I kept moving: _____
_____
_____

What I drank: _____
_____

Did I need a "Quick Fix" today? _____

A Victorian Breakfast

Instead of eating breakfast right after exercising, fine Victorian families would sit down to eat after daily prayers. Although this might take the same half hour, the rest of the meal had nothing to do with the 5-Day Miracle Diet—or any healthier diet, for that matter:

A fine repast would consist of broiled sheep's kidney, toast and thick butter, eggs, and a concoction called kedgeree, a dish made with fish, rice, hard-boiled eggs, and spices—all heated in heavy cream!

The "miracle" in Victorian times was that families survived long enough for dinner!

● ●

❝It's hard to describe what being in good blood sugar feels like. I mean, I can tell you that I have more energy, that I'm more focused and happier in what I do. But these are only words. And unless you've experienced what I have, it's, well, you can't describe it. You have to get into good blood sugar to know what I mean.❞

— A forty-nine-year-old salesman and father of two

● ●

> *"The 5-Day Miracle Diet makes you an active participant in life. Suddenly, you speak up and make decisions!"*
>
> **—The Daily Adele Dose**

• •

Date:

What I ate...for breakfast: _____
_____
_____

What I ate...for my morning hard-chew snacks: _____
_____

What I ate...for lunch: _____
_____
_____
_____

What I ate...for my afternoon soft chews: _____

What I ate...for dinner: _____
_____
_____
_____

How I felt: _____
_____
_____

How I kept moving: _____
_____
_____

What I drank: _____
_____

Did I eat an unsweetened cereal today? _____

Special Grilled Vegetables

When I envision grilled vegetables, I can't believe that they're not fattening! They are so delicious, so colorful, and so crunchy that it's difficult to comprehend that they have so few calories, even if you add in a drizzle of oil! I prefer these on the barbecue, but you can make them in your broiler and they'll be just as scrumptious.

What you'll need:
Marinade
- 2 tablespoons chopped onion
- 2 tablespoons chopped garlic (optional)
- 2 tablespoons chopped parsley
- 2 tablespoons chopped chives
- Juice of 1 lemon
- 2 tablespoons extra-virgin olive oil
- Salt and pepper to taste

- 16 slices eggplant (preferably Italian), sliced ¼ inch thick
- 16 slices zucchini, sliced ¼ inch thick
- 8 slices tomatoes (omit if using outdoor or stovetop grill), sliced ¼ inch thick
- 8 slices onion, sliced ¼ inch thick
- 8 large whole asparagus
- 16 large mushroom caps
- 8 large endives, cut in half lengthwise, blanched by boiling in water for 2 minutes
- 2 red bell peppers, cut into 4 pieces

What you'll do:
Mix the marinade ingredients together. Add the vegetables. Cover with foil or plastic wrap and marinate at room temperature for one hour, stirring occasionally.

If using a broiler:
Preheat the broiler. Lay all vegetables flat on a nonstick or sprayed baking sheet. Turn the oven temperature down to 400°F. Place the baking sheet in the oven and cook until tops of veggies are light brown.

If using an outdoor barbecue or stovetop grill:
Light the fire. When the grill is getting hot, place the vegetables in wire baskets. Put the baskets on the grill and barbecue until light brown.

Serves 4. Don't forget to add the oil to your daily fat allotment.

> **"Timing is everything! It's what makes this diet uniquely successful!"**
>
> —*The Daily Adele Dose*

● ●

Date:

What I ate...for breakfast: _____
_____
_____

What I ate...for my morning hard-chew snacks: _____
_____

What I ate...for lunch: _____
_____
_____
_____

What I ate...for my afternoon soft chews: _____

What I ate...for dinner: _____
_____
_____
_____

How I felt: _____
_____
_____

How I kept moving: _____
_____
_____

What I drank: _____
_____

Did I ask my dinner host for the specific veggies I needed in my crudités? _____

A WEEKLY SHOPPING LIST

Here's a basic list of some of the foods you'll need every week on the 5-Day Miracle Diet. Mix and match your hard-chew choices. You can purchase these once a week at the store, storing the fresh produce in perforated bags. Fill in what you need on a quick stop during the week. And buy your fish fresh from the store the day you eat it.

The Basic 5-Day Miracle Diet Grocery List

- 12 firm, fresh apples
- 1 bag of string beans (six handfuls in a bag)
- 1 pound bag of baby carrots or organic full-grown carrots
- 1 head of red cabbage
- 2 packages of free-range chicken breasts, skinned and boned
- 1 package of tofu
- ½ dozen eggs
- 2 small cans tuna, packed in spring water
- 18 (1-liter) bottles of water
- 1 head of broccoli
- 1 head of cauliflower
- 1 package naturally cooked sliced turkey
- 3 oranges
- 1 bunch asparagus
- 1 package low-fat cheese
- 1 jar natural peanut butter
- 1 loaf whole-grain bread
- 1 package couscous
- 1 package rice
- 3 Idaho potatoes for baking
- 1 bottle laundry detergent (well, you do have to wash your clothes!)

"If you're a food sensualist like me, you'll eventually need to tailor your diet to appeal to your senses. Dig into your 'Food You Adore.' Relish the whole-grain bread. Drink your water sparkling cold. Be passionate. It's the only way you'll 'own' the 5-Day Miracle Diet!"

—*The Daily Adele Dose*

• •

Date:

What I ate...for breakfast: _____

_____

_____

What I ate...for my morning hard-chew snacks: _____

_____

What I ate...for lunch: _____

_____

_____

_____

What I ate...for my afternoon soft chews: _____

What I ate...for dinner: _____

_____

_____

_____

How I felt: _____

_____

_____

How I kept moving: _____

_____

_____

What I drank: _____

_____

Did I set the table for my solo dinner tonight, complete with flowers?

_____

RED SNAPPER
CRAZY WATER

The first time I tasted this dish, I
felt as if I were out in the Southwest,
eating a divine dish in a clay-red adobe. It is
exotic, but very much an American dish. Use only fresh snapper for a
taste that's heavenly. And make sure your sparkling water is just opened
for optimum freshness. Serve with freshly steamed brown rice and a tricolored salad mixed with one of my three dressings (which you'll find
within these pages) and you, too, can close your eyes and be under a
star-studded Southwestern sky!

What you'll need:

24 ounces red snapper fillet
 4 sliced plum (Roma) tomatoes
 8 sliced garlic cloves
 8 basil leaves
 2 tablespoons chopped parsley
½ teaspoon crushed red pepper
 2 cups sparkling bottled water
    Salt and pepper to taste

What you'll do:

Place the red snapper fillets in the bottom of a flat roasting pan. Mix all
the rest of the ingredients together and sprinkle over the fish. Boil for 15
minutes.

Serves 4 (male-sized portions). Women: Slice off about 2 ounces of fish
and put aside. Wrap in foil and eat for breakfast or add to lunch or dinner the next day.

"When I'm in bad blood sugar, restaurant Chinese noodles frantically wave hello. When I'm in good blood sugar, they lie there, powerless, boring, and begging to be whisked away by the waiter."

—The Daily Adele Dose

• •

Date:

What I ate...for breakfast: _____
_____
_____

What I ate...for my morning hard-chew snacks: _____
_____

What I ate...for lunch: _____
_____
_____
_____

What I ate...for my afternoon soft chews: _____

What I ate...for dinner: _____
_____
_____
_____

How I felt: _____
_____
_____

How I kept moving: _____
_____
_____

What I drank: _____
_____

Did I drink at least eight glasses of water? _____

FISH OUT OF WATER

As anyone who has read my book or heard me speak knows, I love fish. Personally, I think it's a "miracle" food, and it's certainly a staple of the 5-Day Miracle Diet. It has the right kind of fatty oil (and the fat it does have is essential to life!) and few calories—plus it packs a whole lot of nutrients in one portion.

But I've found in my practice that many people are afraid of fish. They don't know how to cook it. They don't know when it's been cooked enough. And most of all, they haven't a clue how to make it taste good!

✔ Here's a secret! Find a store that sells really fresh fish. The fresher the fish, the better-tasting. The person behind the counter will always be happy to clean and fillet your fish, if you ask. Don't be shy. Ask away! It makes cooking easier.

✔ You can recognize fresh fish by their eyes. They are clear and bright, not cloudy.

✔ Fish is cooked when the flesh is no longer translucent and it easily flakes when tested with a fork. Don't overcook. If you don't like fish, it's probably because you've always had it cooked too long. It becomes dry, tough, and tasteless.

✔ Grilling, poaching, and broiling fish are all low-calorie staple methods of the "fish cook." Add some seasonings, such as herbes de Provence, Italian spices, or a drop of garlic or mustard powder. Sprinkle with lemon and a drizzle of olive oil for moisture. Add some veggies in the same pot, grill, or broiler, and within minutes you have lunch or dinner!

"Accept the fact that what you see reflected in the mirror is not at all what others see. Who knows? They might even see someone fabulous!"

—*The Daily Adele Dose*

• •

Date:

What I ate...for breakfast: _____
_____
_____

What I ate...for my morning hard-chew snacks: _____
_____

What I ate...for lunch: _____
_____
_____
_____

What I ate...for my afternoon soft chews: _____

What I ate...for dinner: _____
_____
_____
_____

How I felt: _____
_____
_____

How I kept moving: _____
_____
_____

What I drank: _____
_____

Did I take my calcium/magnesium supplement? _____

WEEKLY ASSESSMENT

WEIGHTY ISSUES

Last week's weight: _____

Pounds lost: _____

New weight: _____

Don't forget those lost ounces and half pounds. They add up!

• •

Eat consciously and sensuously. Enjoy the color, the texture, the smell, and, of course, the taste! Believe it or not, you'll eat less.

• •

A WEEK'S "POCKETFUL OF MIRACLES"

What I like best about this section is that it gets you to think. It gets you to look at your life and *appreciate* what you have—and where you're going. It's sort of like the cliché "stopping to smell the roses."

And tell me, isn't it better to see the world in a positive way? It's just as real to see the miracles in life as it is to see the despair. In some ways, you have to look *harder* to find the joy. You sometimes have to take a risk and stand out from the crowd.

The 5-Day Miracle Diet is the facilitator. It helps you see the best there is out there—and *do* the best that you can without fear!

Here's a miracle that I found an act of both kindness and courage, one a reader sent me:

• *When I began the 5-Day Miracle Diet, I just knew it was the right program for me, and I wanted to share it with a friend who's very sensitive about her weight. I couldn't let this opportunity to help her pass, even if it meant she might be angry.*

Now it's your turn: _____

_____

_____

"There's nothing like the feeling of being in good blood sugar. It's, well, a miracle!"

—*The Daily Adele Dose*

• •

Date:

What I ate...for breakfast: _____
_____
_____

What I ate...for my morning hard-chew snacks: _____
_____

What I ate...for lunch: _____
_____
_____
_____

What I ate...for my afternoon soft chews: _____

What I ate...for dinner:_____
_____
_____
_____

How I felt: _____
_____
_____

How I kept moving: _____
_____
_____

What I drank: _____
_____

Did I take up something new in my life, like an art class or gardening?
_____

Reward the Good Fight

Last week, an attractive, successful client of mine said, "I'd been struggling with my weight so long I felt like a failure."

I understood. I understood the confusion people have between struggle and failure. Somehow, they get it into their minds that the everyday attempts, the determination to keep going—which is the struggle—is the same as failure, because they aren't reaching their goal.

How can trying to do better or work harder or hurdle through something be called failure? It doesn't make sense!

And yet many of my clients, working hard at their goals and achieving things in their everyday life, act as though they were total washouts!

The only true failure occurs when you quit. If you stop, you fail.

But struggle is not quitting—not by a long shot.

Struggle needs to be rewarded. If you are struggling, be nice to yourself. Be proud. You're working hard at something you want to achieve.

"Believe it or not, once you've begun my diet, you'll crave less salt and less caffeine. You just won't want these 'fixes' anymore."

—*The Daily Adele Dose*

• •

Date:

What I ate...for breakfast: _____
_____
_____

What I ate...for my morning hard-chew snacks: _____
_____

What I ate...for lunch: _____
_____
_____
_____

What I ate...for my afternoon soft chews: _____

What I ate...for dinner: _____
_____
_____
_____

How I felt: _____
_____
_____

How I kept moving: _____
_____
_____

What I drank: _____
_____

Did I taste my food before shaking salt on it? _____

WINTER WHITE OMELET

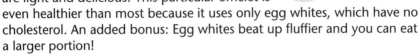

An omelet is a wonderful canvas to which you can add any number of colors, from vegetables to herbs. Omelets are light and delicious. This particular omelet is even healthier than most because it uses only egg whites, which have no cholesterol. An added bonus: Egg whites beat up fluffier and you can eat a larger portion!

What you'll need:
2   tablespoons extra-virgin olive oil (optional)
1   cup raw vegetables, finely chopped. Choose any combination of the following: spinach, onions, broccoli, peppers, scallions, leeks, asparagus, tomatoes, zucchini, mushrooms (any variety), arugula, watercress, Brussels sprouts, escarole, peas
4   egg whites
    Salt and pepper to taste

What you'll do:
If using oil:
   Heat the oil in a medium skillet and sauté the chopped vegetables for 5 minutes, stirring constantly.
   Beat the egg whites with a whisk until frothy. Add salt and pepper to the egg whites and stir in the vegetables.
   Heat an 8-inch nonstick skillet until drops of water sizzle in it. Lower the heat to medium and cook each side of the omelet for 2 minutes.

If not using oil:
   Steam the vegetables until only slightly crunchy. Set aside.
   Beat the egg whites with a whisk until frothy. Add salt and pepper to the egg whites. Stir the vegetables into the egg whites.
   Heat an 8-inch nonstick skillet until drops of water sizzle in it. Lower the heat to medium and cook the omelet on each side for 2 minutes.

Serves 1. If using the oil version, add to your daily fat allotment accordingly.

MIRACLE DIET CHEF'S HINT: When sautéing foods in a skillet, you can either use a drop of oil (but don't forget to add it to your fat allotment!), a nonstick pan, or olive oil Pam spray—it's even lower in calories and it tastes good!

"Just five days on my diet plan and hope becomes more than a glimmer. It is a real possibility!"

—The Daily Adele Dose

• •

Date:

What I ate...for breakfast: _____
_____
_____

What I ate...for my morning hard-chew snacks: _____
_____

What I ate...for lunch: _____
_____
_____
_____

What I ate...for my afternoon soft chews: _____

What I ate...for dinner: _____
_____
_____
_____

How I felt: _____
_____
_____

How I kept moving: _____
_____
_____

What I drank: _____
_____

Did I sleep in this weekend—and correctly compensate for my breakfast, lunch, and hard chews? _____

A STEAK-AND-POTATOES KINDA GUY

Sometimes nothing will do the trick but one of those old-fashioned, mahogany-walled, white-tableclothed pubs, the kinds of places that are reminiscent of "old New York" (or Chicago, Detroit, San Francisco—you name it).

You'd think that the only healthy item on display was the pepper! Wrong. You *can* go to a chop house and enjoy yourself (without feeling you've gone back fifty years, to when red meat, beer, butter, and fried anything were thought to be as healthy as a Red Delicious apple!). Here are some hints if you decide to join your colleagues after work for supper in a pub:

✔ One thing about these places: they make *great* burgers. As long as they're broiled, go for—half! Take the other half home, freeze, and use for lunch or dinner's protein one day the following week. And don't forget to pile on the veggies: tomato, onion, lettuce. Yum! You won't even notice the fact that there's less burger on your bun.

✔ And speaking of bun, it's usually made of refined white flour. You're better off without it.

✔ Try not to use ketchup. It has sugar. Try mustard instead. It gives burgers a piquant flavor!

✔ Fill up on salad. Eat yours with plenty of balsamic vinegar or dressing on the side.

✔ Whenever possible, choose an appetizer over an entrée. (Main dishes tend to be too plentiful in steak houses.)

Dishes you can really sink your teeth into—without adding fat, sugar, and calories!
✔ Shrimp cocktail or oysters and a large house salad
✔ A plain baked potato and grilled chicken
✔ Steamed lobster sprinkled with fresh lemon (forget the butter sauce!)
✔ Grilled veggies
✔ Flank steak or top round instead of porterhouse. There's less fat.

When only a burger will do, try these hearty "Extras"—as little as possible but enough to make you happy. Cheers!
✔ A juicy burger topped with a Bermuda onion—with the roll
✔ A house salad made with chunky Roquefort dressing
✔ Steak fries

"You need to love yourself first, before you can love any-one else, before you can change the way you live. You need to feel you deserve to feel good!"

—The Daily Adele Dose

• •

Date:

What I ate...for breakfast: _____
_____
_____

What I ate...for my morning hard-chew snacks: _____
_____

What I ate...for lunch: _____
_____
_____
_____

What I ate...for my afternoon soft chews: _____

What I ate...for dinner: _____
_____
_____
_____

How I felt: _____
_____
_____

How I kept moving: _____
_____
_____

What I drank: _____
_____

Did I buy a new exercise outfit or gear to help me get moving?
_____

A BIRTHDAY GIFT FOR A FORTY-YEAR-OLD WOMAN AND THE STORY THAT WILL STAY WITH ME FOREVER

I was on a book tour for *The 5-Day Miracle Diet* and was waiting in the airport for my plane home. There was still about fifteen minutes to go before my departure, and I was relaxing in a chair watching the planes take off outside the window. I was startled out of my reverie when I looked up and noticed an overweight woman standing next to me. She grasped a copy of my book in her hands, which were crossed in front of her chest. She coughed. "It's you!" she said, pointing to my picture on the cover.

I smiled at her. "Would you like me to sign that book for you?" I asked her.

She hesitated. She didn't want to bother me....

I gently told her it was absolutely no bother. I was waiting for my plane, after all.

The woman smiled. We began to talk about the 5-Day Miracle Diet. She told me that she'd been on it for seven days and had already lost weight. "I couldn't believe it. I actually woke up this morning and took a walk! And I wasn't even out of breath."

I told her that that was terrific. Then she told me that tomorrow was her forty-first birthday. "What a fabulous gift to give yourself!" I exclaimed.

The woman just looked at me and burst into tears. "I have hope. You saved my life."

I instinctively hugged her. She hugged me back.

I will never forget that woman and the great gift she gave me—and herself.

"Most of us live in low blood sugar. But not you! You have the 5-Day Miracle Diet to change all that!"

—*The Daily Adele Dose*

• •

Date:

What I ate...for breakfast: _____
_____
_____

What I ate...for my morning hard-chew snacks: _____
_____

What I ate...for lunch: _____
_____
_____
_____

What I ate...for my afternoon soft chews: _____

What I ate...for dinner: _____
_____
_____
_____

How I felt: _____
_____
_____

How I kept moving: _____
_____
_____

What I drank: _____
_____

Did I take my vitamins with a full glass of water? _____

SEE YOUR CEREAL

What you see isn't always what you get. Those cereal boxes that line your shelf might look healthy, but in reality they can wreak havoc on your blood-sugar balance. Look at the labels. You might be surprised.

SUBTLE SUGAR BABY CHOICES:

Cheerios
Rice Chex
Special K
Corn Flakes
All-Bran
Kix
All Healthy Choice brand cereals

Believe it or not, all these cereals contain some sugar, just enough to keep your cravings strong and your blood sugar bad—even when eaten on alternate days.

5-DAY MIRACLE DIET CHOICES:

Bran Flakes
Puffed Wheat
Puffed Rice
Shredded Wheat
Wheat Chex
Wheat germ (3 tablespoons)
All Grainfields brand cereals, except those with raisins

"Fat is essential to life—so is good taste. But a small amount goes far."

—*The Daily Adele Dose*

● ●

Date:

What I ate...for breakfast: _____
_____
_____

What I ate...for my morning hard-chew snacks: _____
_____

What I ate...for lunch: _____
_____
_____
_____

What I ate...for my afternoon soft chews: _____

What I ate...for dinner: _____
_____
_____
_____

How I felt: _____
_____
_____

How I kept moving: _____
_____
_____

What I drank: _____
_____

Did I take my fat allotment into account when I followed a recipe?
_____

> **"What is food to one man may be fierce poison to others."**
>
> —*Lucretius (95–55 B.C.)*

IT'S GREEK TO ME

They might have created the gyro and baklava later, but the early Greeks were pure in heart—and stomach. Both rich and poor ate a modest diet—and except for the double dose of wine, a fairly healthy one by today's standards. Both breakfast and lunch were a simple crust of bread dipped in wine. Dinner held more bread, this time with goat cheese, beans, cabbage, and fish. Dessert was fruit and nuts.

The Greeks liked meat, but only on feast days. For meat lovers, this would truly be a "hard chew" to swallow.

"Just think: This time it is really going to happen. This time you are going to lose weight and feel better than you ever have in your life!"

—The Daily Adele Dose

• •

Date:

What I ate...for breakfast: _____

_____

_____

What I ate...for my morning hard-chew snacks: _____

_____

What I ate...for lunch: _____

_____

_____

_____

What I ate...for my afternoon soft chews: _____

What I ate...for dinner: _____

_____

_____

_____

How I felt: _____

_____

_____

How I kept moving: _____

_____

_____

What I drank: _____

_____

Did I try tofu as a protein choice? _____

WEEKLY ASSESSMENT

WEIGHTY ISSUES

Last week's weight: _____

Pounds lost: _____

New weight: _____

Don't forget those lost ounces and half pounds. They add up!

• •

**Remember, no one got fat eating one potato chip,
one cookie, or one big serving of pasta. If you've "succumbed,"
enjoy it—and keep going on the 5-Day Miracle Diet.**

• •

A WEEK'S "POCKETFUL OF MIRACLES"

"*T*he Times, They Are A-Changin' " is a classic song by Bob Dylan (which you might not know if you're not a Baby Boomer). He was talking about protests and rebellion and growing up during the sixties.

But we're not talking protest here in 5-Day Miracle Diet land. We're talking health.

Think about it. Don't you have more energy than you did before you started the diet? Do you have a glow to your cheeks? A more confident air? These are all miracles, every single one of them. They might not bring world peace, but they will bring peace of mind to you.

Here's a sign of the times "miracle" a client told me with tears in her eyes:

• *I thought I was ready for retirement at work. In fact, I'd even made an appointment with my accountant to see if it was feasible. But ever since I started your diet, I've had more strength and vitality than I ever had— even in my youth. I've given retirement the shaft, at least for now. There's too much I want to accomplish at work, and I have the energy to do it.*

Now it's your turn: _____

_____

_____

"If you are in good blood sugar, those daily uncontrollable cravings will be gone—and you can enjoy a fabulous 'Food You Adore'!"

—The Daily Adele Dose

• •

Date:

What I ate...for breakfast: _____

_____

_____

What I ate...for my morning hard-chew snacks: _____

_____

What I ate...for lunch: _____

_____

_____

_____

What I ate...for my afternoon soft chews: _____

What I ate...for dinner: _____

_____

_____

_____

How I felt: _____

_____

_____

How I kept moving: _____

_____

_____

What I drank: _____

_____

Did I try popcorn without butter at the movies? _____

ELLA'S CHICKEN PITA

Tired of the usual salad or sliced turkey and bread for lunch? Try this delicious and original alternative...named after one of the finest chefs on Long Island! It's made with acorn squash and chicken, and it's so scrumptious you may never go back to regular sandwiches again!

What you'll need:

  2   teaspoons oil, preferably canola or extra-virgin olive
 16   ounces skinless, boneless chicken breasts
  8   ounces acorn squash, peeled
      Salt and pepper to taste
  4   teaspoons lemon juice
  2   teaspoons Dijon mustard
      Pinch of chopped parsley
  1   sliced plum (Roma) tomato, seeds removed
  2   tablespoons chopped celery
  2   tablespoons chopped carrots
  4   mini pitas, whole-wheat, if possible
      Chopped tomato, for garnish (optional)
      Shredded lettuce, for garnish (optional)

What you'll do:

Heat the oil in a small skillet until a drop of water sizzles in its center. Sauté the chicken breasts until light brown, about 5 minutes. Cut the chicken into medium chunks and let cool.

Cut the acorn squash into chunks. Boil enough lightly salted water to cover the squash. Add the squash and boil for 20 minutes, until soft. Drain and let cool.

Place 4 ounces of the chicken, the acorn squash, ¾ cup water, and the lemon juice, mustard, parsley, tomato, salt, and pepper in a blender or food processor. Blend for 3 minutes.

Remove the mixture from the blender and add the celery and carrots. Toss with the remaining chicken.

Fill the pita pockets with the chicken mixture. Add the chopped tomatoes and/or shredded lettuce to the pita, if desired.

Serves 4. Men: Add 1 ounce low-fat sliced cheese to your salad. Don't forget to add the squash to your starchy carbohydrate total.

"The diet is all about making it your own!"

—*The Daily Adele Dose*

• •

Date:

What I ate...for breakfast: _____
_____
_____

What I ate...for my morning hard-chew snacks: _____
_____

What I ate...for lunch: _____
_____
_____
_____

What I ate...for my afternoon soft chews: _____

What I ate...for dinner: _____
_____
_____
_____

How I felt: _____
_____
_____

How I kept moving: _____
_____
_____

What I drank: _____
_____

Did I discover a new appropriate food for myself? _____

"OH, HOW I HATE TO WAKE UP IN THE MORNING"

Judy was a worrier—and a longtime client of mine. Over the months together, we've learned a lot about each other. Judy has lost twenty pounds, but it was almost an afterthought. She really came to me because she felt tired and had lost her joie de vivre; she was...worried.

It was no wonder Judy felt ill. She was in bad blood sugar, creating a chemical imbalance that caused her lack of energy and focus. It made her hair lank and her skin pale. And it created cravings that made her eat all the wrong things—a vicious cycle that had to be stopped...immediately.

Judy began the 5-Day Miracle Diet, and it changed everything. Within days, she found the vitality she thought she'd lost. Within weeks, she had gained confidence and a poised, new look. But the best news was what she told me last week:

"You know me, Adele. I wake up every morning worried. It's my *fathead* hat. Not even the diet could stop it! I keep thinking about what I have to do, how I'm going to do it, even what I'm going to wear...except today was different, really different."

She paused, grinning at me. She couldn't wait to tell me what had happened. "I still woke up the same way, all worried and stuff, but this time I actually told myself to stop. Just get up and go through the day, Judy. Don't worry about anything. Let the day happen."

Judy clapped her hands. "That's just what I did. It was fine. I mean, I didn't get a promotion or anything, but nothing bad happened either. I stayed on the diet, I ate my hard chews, I went to my meetings, just like always. But I wasn't worried. Not anymore. *Let the day happen*. It's become my mantra."

"Owning" the diet doesn't come as a startling epiphany. It isn't an "Ohmigod, where has this been all my life!" kind of thing. "Owning" the 5-Day Miracle Diet comes from living every day in good blood sugar. It comes from writing in your journal and determining your *fathead* issues, your vulnerable times, and the times when you feel empowered.

It comes from situations like this one, like Judy waking up and deciding to just let the day happen.

"Owning" the diet can happen to you, too, if you let it happen.

"After cope, cope, and more cope, there is hope!"
— *The Daily Adele Dose*

• •

Date:

What I ate...for breakfast: _____
_____
_____

What I ate...for my morning hard-chew snacks: _____
_____

What I ate...for lunch: _____
_____
_____
_____

What I ate...for my afternoon soft chews: _____

What I ate...for dinner: _____
_____
_____
_____

How I felt: _____
_____
_____

How I kept moving: _____
_____
_____

What I drank: _____
_____

Did I choose a "Food You Adore" "Extra" in good blood sugar? _____

I SAY CHINESE, PLEASE

Eating in a Chinese restaurant doesn't have to be a thing of the past if you're on the 5-Day Miracle Diet. Remember, it's a lifestyle plan, not a diet you go on and off like a roller-coaster ride. That means eating anything you decide—and dining out at least twice a week in restaurants you always enjoyed.

Chinese restaurants are very popular—and with good reason. They're inexpensive and the food tastes great. Sure, there's a lot of fat in many of the dishes, but not all. Here are some suggestions to make your visit to your local Chinese take-out restaurant an "un-exotic" experience:

1. Unless you're in terrific blood sugar, ask the waiter to take away the noodles. If you've read *The 5-Day Miracle Diet*, you know how deadly they can be!
2. Steamed vegetables and tofu or seafood and chicken dishes are recommended, but you *are* free to have an occasional meat entrée. It's allowed!
3. Add flavor with Chinese mustard or choose your sauce the way you like it: *sans oil*, as a dipping sauce of soy, garlic, and ginger; *with oil*, as a favorite dipping sauce, or *as a sauce on the dish itself* (using chopsticks to wipe off excess sauce from each tender morsel on the side of your plate). It's up to you. After all, *you* "own" the diet and *you* can decide how to control the amount of fat you consume.
4. One of my favorites is Lake Tung Shrimp, a popular dish made with shrimp, snow pea pods, and broccoli in a light white sauce. I eat only half the entrée and I skip the rice. It's satisfying and delicious, but don't be deceived by the broccoli. Once it's cooked, it's not enough of a hard chew to count. So make sure you eat your hard-chew snack *before* you get to the restaurant.
5. If possible, order steamed brown rice instead of white rice. It's healthier.
6. Opt for tea without sugar and, for optimum benefits and no caffeine, ice-cold water is always available (and it's free!).

Some delectable classic Chinese temptations that make Imperial "Extras":

✔ An egg roll or spring roll
✔ Fried rice (even the House Special Fried Rice!)
✔ Orange beef, sesame chicken, and any other entrée made with sauce
✔ Kwang pao dishes (made with peanuts and hot sauce)
✔ Chow fun and lo mein dishes
✔ A fortune cookie

"Think before you go for the 'light.' It's not always right!"

—*The Daily Adele Dose*

• •

Date:

What I ate...for breakfast: _____
_____
_____

What I ate...for my morning hard-chew snacks: _____
_____

What I ate...for lunch: _____
_____
_____
_____

What I ate...for my afternoon soft chews: _____

What I ate...for dinner: _____
_____
_____
_____

How I felt: _____
_____
_____

How I kept moving: _____
_____
_____

What I drank: _____
_____

Did I have breakfast within a half hour of getting up or exercising?
_____

Hello, Hello, Carbo Lovers Everywhere!

As you know, the 5-Day Miracle Diet is not about sacrifice. I don't want you to feel miserable, deprived because you can't eat your pasta or your bagel. I want you to feel fabulous *because your face is no longer bloated, because your stomach is flat, because your vitality, strength, and boundless energy are back.*

That's what stripping the carbs *will do. Once your body is in good blood sugar, you'll be able to* strip *easily and quickly (even without the help of Demi Moore). Within days, those cravings for carbs will cease to exist.*

You'll find the steps you'll need to do in The 5-Day Miracle Diet. *Once you've stabilized your body,* stripping the carbs *becomes a way of life. And guess what. You can still have your rice or beans every third night—and pasta once a week (if you* really *still need it!). You can even try the fabulous pasta recipe you'll find in the pages of this book. And if you find it's hard to come back after a pasta night, make it a "Food You Adore"—along with your bagels.*

See, you never lose your pastas and other carbs. You simply learn how *to eat them—and when!*

"The longer you're on the 5-Day Miracle Diet, the smaller detours will be—and the more the wonderful feelings of empowerment and well-being will soar! "

—*The Daily Adele Dose*

• •

Date:

What I ate...for breakfast: _____

_____

_____

What I ate...for my morning hard-chew snacks: _____

_____

What I ate...for lunch: _____

_____

_____

_____

What I ate...for my afternoon soft chews: _____

What I ate...for dinner: _____

_____

_____

_____

How I felt: _____

_____

_____

How I kept moving: _____

_____

_____

What I drank: _____

_____

Did I take the time to enjoy my meals? _____

ASPARAGUS FROMAGE

This unusual side dish is a wonderful accompaniment for just about anything: roasted chicken, sliced tenderloin, lamb, or one of my delicious fish dishes. It is quick and easy to prepare and can be used for lunch or dinner. You can enjoy one serving sans guilt, because the 23 calories' worth of grated Parmesan cheese will not impact on your 5-Day Miracle Diet. Bon appétit!

What you'll need:

24 large asparagus
 1 tablespoon salt (reduce amount if you are limiting salt for health reasons)
 4 tablespoons freshly grated Parmesan cheese
 8 cups water

What you'll do:

Preheat the oven to 450°F.

Bring 8 cups water and salt to a roaring boil in a large pot or asparagus pan. While the water is coming to a boil, wash the asparagus and discard the white bottoms. Place the asparagus in the boiling water for 5 minutes. Strain in a colander. Cool the asparagus under running cold water.

Place four groups of asparagus (six stalks in each group) flat on a baking sheet. Lightly sprinkle 1 tablespoon Parmesan cheese over each bundle. Put the baking sheet under the broiler and immediately turn to broil. Broil the asparagus for approximately 60 seconds, until light brown. WATCH CAREFULLY to make sure they do not burn.

Remove the baking sheet and let asparagus cool for 2 minutes. Serve hot.

Serves 4.

MIRACLE DIET CHEF'S HINT: Using the best Parmesan cheese is what makes this recipe so fabulous—and brings out its incredible taste. The Parmesan used in all the finest restaurants is Parmigiano-Reggiano. You can purchase it either in a block or already grated.

"You can't fail on the 5-Day Miracle Diet. All you can do is learn!"

—*The Daily Adele Dose*

• •

Date:

What I ate...for breakfast: _____

_____

_____

What I ate...for my morning hard-chew snacks: _____

_____

What I ate...for lunch: _____

_____

_____

_____

What I ate...for my afternoon soft chews: _____

What I ate...for dinner: _____

_____

_____

_____

How I felt: _____

_____

_____

How I kept moving: _____

_____

_____

What I drank: _____

_____

Did I stop eating for the day after dinner? _____

"Before I started this diet, I felt out of control. Nothing made me happy. I didn't want to go out. I didn't want to see people. I was ashamed of myself. I felt **terrible.** *No more. I've only lost ten pounds so far, but what a difference it makes. I stand up tall now. I feel good seeing my friends. And I even laugh now. A real, rich, hearty laugh. Could this all be good blood sugar? Wow. It really is a miracle."*

—A housewife and mother of three in the suburbs

"To lead a full, vital life you need to be healthy. The 5-Day Miracle Diet provides the good foods and the body chemistry to ensure that great life!"

—*The Daily Adele Dose*

● ●

Date:

What I ate...for breakfast: _____
_____
_____

What I ate...for my morning hard-chew snacks: _____
_____

What I ate...for lunch: _____
_____
_____
_____

What I ate...for my afternoon soft chews: _____

What I ate...for dinner: _____
_____
_____
_____

How I felt: _____
_____
_____

How I kept moving: _____
_____
_____

What I drank: _____
_____

Did I remember to bring my water to work? _____

N o! Is it really a whole month! I am so excited for you because I know exactly how you feel if you've been sticking to the program: fabulous! From someone who's been there and back, I know you are probably saying, "It couldn't possibly be another month. It was too easy. Too simple. In terms of energy, health, concentration, memory, flexibility, strength—well, you name it—I feel great!" You might add, as countless numbers of my clients have, "This diet has changed my whole life."

Or maybe, like other clients, you might be saying, "I could do better. I need to reassess." Perhaps this has been a tougher month than usual. Maybe the *fathead* reared its ugly profile a bit too often. Maybe you were tempted by too many foods at too many affairs. Or your blood sugar wasn't as good as it could be.

How to get back on track? Simple. Start with your journal. See where temptation might have been lurking. Check to see if you ate the right foods in the right combination at the right times. It's all here. Within these pages, in good old black-and-white.

To separate fact from "fat"asy, start with some bottom-line proof of your progress to keep that motivation strong: the way your clothes fit, the way you move, and the way you feel now—four months later!

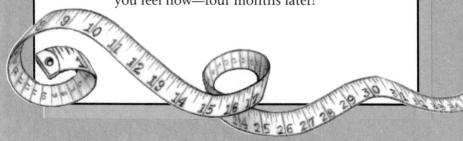

Inch-by-Inch

Bust/chest: _____   Upper arms: _____

Wrists: _____   Waist: _____

Abdomen: _____   Hips and buttocks: _____

IN A WORD...

Sum up your monthly experience in one or two words. Use it as your "mantra" in the month to come. It's easy now that you've made the 5-Day Miracle Diet yours to keep! Here's one of my favorites:

I'm living my life—and loving it!

What's your good word?

_____

Shout it out. You should feel proud!

Have you ever noticed the number of fattening food phrases we have in our culture today? "Easy as pie." "A piece of cake." "Whipped cream with a cherry on top." Fight back! Eat "an apple a day"—and carrots, string beans, and cauliflower, too!

Remember, in these hectic times, it's important to stop and reflect on the 3 "R's":

1. **Regroup** the foods you eat and your eating schedule. 2. **Rethink** the way you eat—and why. 3. **Replenish** your body and soul with nurturing, nutrient-rich foods.

WEEKLY ASSESSMENT

WEIGHTY ISSUES

Last week's weight: _____

Pounds lost: _____

New weight: _____

Don't forget those lost ounces and half pounds. They add up!

• •

Feeling stressed-out and needing to run to the fridge? Try jumping in a lake—or a pool or even the shower—to cool off. It's much lower in calories—and it's good for you, too!

• •

A WEEK'S "POCKETFUL OF MIRACLES"

*H*ere's a hypothetical situation, but one that, if not this week, will presumably occur during the months you are on the 5-Day Miracle Diet: You've had a miserable week. Yes. It's true. Murphy's Law sometimes comes true: Whatever can go wrong will go wrong! In short, this is a week you'd rather forget. And right about now, your *fathead* is probably making noises, urging you to sabotage your good "blood-sugar" efforts.The last thing you want to do is think of a miracle from last week! And yet it is probably the most important thing you can do. It will keep you going and put you back on a course that moves in a positive direction.

So think of these words, spoken by one of my clients. They will help you get through the bad times:
• *I had a miserable day, and all I could think about was that bottle of wine in the fridge. But I knew that if I drank it, I'd feel horrible—for at least two more days. I didn't need another problem, I needed a solution. So I stayed with Adele!*

Now it's your turn: _____

_____

_____

"Don't let food be the weapon of choice for you. Better to confront and explain. "

—The Daily Adele Dose

• •

Date:

What I ate...for breakfast: _____

_____

_____

What I ate...for my morning hard-chew snacks: _____

_____

What I ate...for lunch: _____

_____

_____

_____

What I ate...for my afternoon soft chews: _____

What I ate...for dinner: _____

_____

_____

_____

How I felt: _____

_____

_____

How I kept moving: _____

_____

_____

What I drank: _____

_____

Did I choose a healthier outlet to deal with my emotions than food?

_____

THE NEW MANTRA: FAT-FREE

One look at the aisles in your supermarket and you'd think that food companies and consumers alike have found the secret of long life: no fat. It's astonishing to me to see such items as fat-free salad dressing, fat-free "butter" spreads—even fat-free Twinkies! Even foods that never had any fat to begin with, like breads, rice, or pasta, will proclaim "No Fat!"

But here's where the problems begin. Fat tastes good—that's why we eat it. Take away the fat and you have to add something to make a food taste palatable, especially a processed food. So what do manufacturers put into no-fat and low-fat cereal, salad dressings, cookies, peanut butter, and, yes, Twinkies? Sugar! You'll actually find more sugar in these items than in the more natural, normal brands.

And fat-free can be hazardous to your health. If you've read *The 5-Day Miracle Diet*, you know that we need a certain amount of fat in our diet for proper digestion, strong nails, and glowing skin. You also know that our bodies cannot manufacture enough of these essential fatty acids, and we need to get a supply from the foods we eat. If we consistently eat "no-fat," we're doing our bodies more harm than good—not to mention that we're playing with our chemistry because of the extra sugar!

I allow just enough healthful oils to be sure you're getting the essential fatty acids you need. An added plus: delicious food. Just try one of my recipes in this book to see how far one "fat allotment" can take your taste buds!

"Craving anything is not the way to live your life. Staying with the 5-Day Miracle Diet is!"

—*The Daily Adele Dose*

• •

Date:

What I ate...for breakfast: _____
_____
_____

What I ate...for my morning hard-chew snacks: _____
_____

What I ate...for lunch: _____
_____
_____
_____

What I ate...for my afternoon soft chews: _____

What I ate...for dinner: _____
_____
_____
_____

How I felt: _____
_____
_____

How I kept moving: _____
_____
_____

What I drank: _____
_____

Did someone tell me how good I look? _____

WEEKDAY EVENING FEVER

The biggest excuse people have for not exercising?
There's not enough time. Period. I can tell you how
important it is for your health. I can show you how wonderful it will make you feel. I can show you some great
exercises, including my fifteen-minute stretch, and you
still won't do it unless you have the time.

But what if it was something terrific, something you
loved to do? Remember when you were a child. You
couldn't stop moving those growing muscles. You'd run
and leap and jump. There wasn't a ledge that wasn't a
temptation to test your balance, a bicycle that didn't
shout, "Ride me!". There wasn't a pool that didn't beg
you to jump in and splash away.

Get back to that time, to that active inner child, and
you will start exercising. You might even refuse to stop!

The best way to get into the groove? Put some of your
favorite music in the CD player, in the tape deck, or on
that dusty turntable. Listen to the music...and dance.
Start slow. Maybe one or two songs. Build up to a whole
album. That's about forty-five minutes of movement. And
who would call it exercise? Not you!

"Healthy eating does not mean you'll never again eat your bagel or your chocolate cake. It just means making choices!"

—*The Daily Adele Dose*

• •

Date:

What I ate...for breakfast: _____
_____
_____

What I ate...for my morning hard-chew snacks: _____
_____

What I ate...for lunch: _____
_____
_____
_____

What I ate...for my afternoon soft chews: _____

What I ate...for dinner: _____
_____
_____
_____

How I felt: _____
_____
_____

How I kept moving: _____
_____
_____

What I drank: _____
_____

Did I do a relaxation exercise today? _____

• •

"I know this sounds like an ad, but the honest-to-God truth is that I am feeling great—more energetic and just plain fabulous—ever since I put down my bagels and my bananas and reached for your book. Thank you, Adele, for turning my life around!"

—A thirty-two-year-old Midwestern banker

• •

"Believe it or not, when you're in good blood sugar, you simply don't think about food!"

—*The Daily Adele Dose*

● ●

Date:

What I ate...for breakfast: _____

_____

_____

What I ate...for my morning hard-chew snacks: _____

_____

What I ate...for lunch:_____

_____

_____

_____

What I ate...for my afternoon soft chews: _____

What I ate...for dinner:_____

_____

_____

_____

How I felt: _____

_____

_____

How I kept moving: _____

_____

_____

What I drank:_____

_____

*Did I eat a fruit dessert at dinner today?*_____

SWEET POTATO SQUASH

It's always difficult to find new, exciting starchy side dishes at dinnertime. Rice is nice, but sometimes you want more. That's where this scrumptious creation comes in; it's literally a sweet potato "pie" with a crust made from squash. Different, yes! Spectacular, yes again!

What you'll need:
1   tablespoon oil, preferably canola or extra-virgin olive
2   (8-ounce) sweet potatoes, peeled and chopped into crouton-size cubes
1   6-ounce chopped onion
4   chopped scallions
4   chopped basil leaves
1   tablespoon chopped parsley
4   chopped plum (Roma) tomatoes
2   8-inch-long opu squash, cut in half lengthwise, seeds removed
    Salt and pepper to taste
    Nutmeg to taste
    Basil bunch, for garnish

What you'll do:
   Preheat the oven to 400° F. Heat a nonstick skillet until drops of water sizzle in its center. Add the oil, sweet potatoes, onion, scallions, basil, parsley, and tomatoes. Simmer for 10 minutes. Add salt and pepper to taste. Remove from heat.
   Sprinkle salt and pepper and nutmeg to taste in opu squash. Fill the squash halves with the sweet potato mixture. Place in a shallow pan or on a baking sheet and bake "squash pies" for 45 minutes.

Serve with a basil bunch stuck into the tip of the squash, for garnish.

Serves 4. Don't forget to add the oil to your daily fat allotment.

MIRACLE DIET CHEF'S HINT: Opu squash is a gourmet's choice for many dishes. It looks like a small acorn squash; it can fit in the palm of your hand! The outside is green with a brown or yellow tint, and it is considered a starchy vegetable.

"You have the power within to change the way you look and feel."

—The Daily Adele Dose

• •

Date:

What I ate...for breakfast: _____
_____
_____

What I ate...for my morning hard-chew snacks: _____
_____

What I ate...for lunch: _____
_____
_____
_____

What I ate...for my afternoon soft chews: _____

What I ate...for dinner: _____
_____
_____
_____

How I felt: _____
_____
_____

How I kept moving: _____
_____
_____

What I drank: _____
_____

Did I ask for my salad dressing on the side? _____

*... And words won't put you in
low blood sugar!*

**"Pleasant words are as a honey-
comb, sweet to the soul, and health
to the bones."**
— *Proverbs 16:24*

You Say Potato, They Say...Disgusting

Okay, so it's not a hard chew or a protein. But it is a wonderful starch to accompany a dinner of veggies and, say, fish. And as a complex carbohydrate, it fills you up for hours.

The simple potato was introduced to America in the sixteenth century. No one knew what to make of them, and most colonists thought they were disgusting. A few fine citizens even blamed them for outbreaks of leprosy and syphilis.

Even in 1720, Americans believed that eating a potato could shorten your life! (Of course, this was discussed at length over beer, buttered mutton, and big fat cigars!)

Today, the spud's rep is solid. As we now know, potatoes make a great starch—sans sour cream, of course!

"I'd no sooner go into my favorite restaurant in low blood sugar than I would go in stark naked!"

—*The Daily Adele Dose*

• •

Date:

What I ate...for breakfast: _____
_____
_____

What I ate...for my morning hard-chew snacks: _____
_____

What I ate...for lunch: _____
_____
_____
_____

What I ate...for my afternoon soft chews: _____

What I ate...for dinner: _____
_____
_____
_____

How I felt: _____
_____
_____

How I kept moving: _____
_____
_____

What I drank: _____
_____

Did I make appropriate choices in a restaurant today? _____

VEGGIE VEGGIE DIP

What I love best about this dip for crudités is that it is made completely with vegetables—kissed with olives and vinegar. It is so divinely piquant that it's given me a whole new slant on vegetable appetizers and snacks. Enjoy your dipping sauce with carrots, cabbage, string beans—whatever you enjoy!

What you'll need:

2 ounces cauliflower florets
3 medium roasted peppers or pimientos
2 tablespoons tarragon vinegar
1 tablespoon white vinegar
3 chopped basil leaves
1 pitted green olive
   Salt and pepper to taste

What you'll do:

   Steam the cauliflower for 2 minutes. Let cool.
   Place all the ingredients, including the cauliflower, into a blender or food processor and blend for 3 minutes.
   Serve in a small cup surrounded by crudités.

Serves 1.

"Feel wonderful!"

—*The Daily Adele Dose*

• •

Date:

What I ate...for breakfast: _____
_____
_____

What I ate...for my morning hard-chew snacks: _____
_____

What I ate...for lunch: _____
_____
_____
_____

What I ate...for my afternoon soft chews: _____

What I ate...for dinner: _____
_____
_____
_____

How I felt: _____
_____
_____

How I kept moving: _____
_____
_____

What I drank: _____
_____

Did I have decaf coffee today? _____

WEIGHTY ISSUES

Last week's weight: _____

Pounds lost: _____

New weight: _____

Don't forget those lost ounces and half pounds. They add up!

• •

When you go to the store for your "vittles," take your time. Think about your purchases before you buy them. It's much easier to walk past the pasta aisle than your kitchen cupboard!

• •

A WEEK'S "POCKETFUL OF MIRACLES"

Wow! Has another week gone by already? At this moment, you may be basking in the glory of your terrific new feeling—and perhaps thinking of some wonderful experiences during the week that will be, if you'll excuse the pun, "a piece of cake"!

Then again, maybe you're a bit discouraged. Your own brand of *fat-head* is talking to you or you are paying too much attention to the scale. All the more reason to think about something special that happened to you this week to recharge those diet batteries.

It doesn't have to be something big to be extraordinary. We don't all have wedding cake to admirably pass up every week!

Here's a little something that packed a big wallop for one of my clients to help jog your memory:

•*I actually walked past my favorite bagel shop on the way to work—and I wasn't even seduced by the aroma! In fact, I had to stop a moment because I didn't get my usual "whiff." I thought I'd walked past the office!*

Now it's your turn: _____

_____

_____

"Stop. Think. Identify and recognize your fathead *problems—and what you think the solutions are."*

—*The Daily Adele Dose*

• •

Date:

What I ate...for breakfast: _____

_____

_____

What I ate...for my morning hard-chew snacks: _____

_____

What I ate...for lunch: _____

_____

_____

_____

What I ate...for my afternoon soft chews: _____

What I ate...for dinner: _____

_____

_____

_____

How I felt: _____

_____

_____

How I kept moving: _____

_____

_____

What I drank: _____

_____

Did I stay within my daily fat allotment? _____

GEARING UP!

One of the reasons many of my clients don't exercise is that they're embarrassed by the way they look in exercise clothes. Although I can reassure them over and over again that nobody's watching, that everybody's too busy looking at themselves in the mirror, it doesn't matter. All they see is fat beneath the latex.

I'd hate for you to be one of my nonaerobic clients just because you don't like the way you look in a leotard or shorts. To help you get past the bumps in order to do the jumps, here are some exercise clothing tips I've found useful in my own life:

The Women's Locker Room

- Buy black leotards and leggings in a size that fits. Many labels, including Gilda and Danskin, have extra-large sizes.
- Stick with leotards with short sleeves and a high neck; you'll be less self-conscious while you jump and turn.
- Oversized T-shirts are a boon. Wear yours over your leotards, knotted at the side for a kick!
- Stay clear of patterns and glitter. Stick with solid colors: leotards, leggings, socks, and exercise shoes all work well in basic black.
- Add a brightly colored "scrunchee" to your hair for a lift!

The Men's Locker Room

- Wear exercise shorts that fit you; a string tie will assure they'll stay up when you jump down.
- Sweatpants hide a multitude of sins. Wear yours in a dark color.
- Wear roomy T-shirts that won't cling to your stomach.
- Add a sweatband around your forehead; it works and it looks smart.
- Ragtag, worn T-shirts might have been cool when you were a teen, but now you're better off with the 100-percent-cotton stretch.

"What is brunch, anyway? Did we invent a fourth meal?"

—*The Daily Adele Dose*

• •

Date:

What I ate...for breakfast: _____
_____
_____

What I ate...for my morning hard-chew snacks: _____
_____

What I ate...for lunch: _____
_____
_____
_____

What I ate...for my afternoon soft chews: _____

What I ate...for dinner: _____
_____
_____
_____

How I felt: _____
_____
_____

How I kept moving: _____
_____
_____

What I drank: _____
_____

Did I smile at myself in the mirror today? _____

A BEDTIME STORY

I remember a story a producer told me during my travels. He was in charge of one of the top morning shows in Canada and he'd come in during the "ten minute call" before show time to give me a spurt of positive energy.

What he told me gave me more than a lift, it made me soar. It turned out that he had a teenage son, a loner, who was about twenty pounds overweight. His son saw my book in the store before I'd even been booked on the show and bought it. During the last month, he'd lost eleven pounds and had, in his proud father's words, "become a changed person." He began to go out with his friends; he met a girl. He actually talked at the dinner table!

When the producer saw what the 5-Day Miracle Diet did for his son, he wanted to try it. "I could stand to lose a few pounds," he laughingly told me. The producer didn't want to take his son's book, he didn't want to discourage him. But there was a problem: There wasn't a copy to be had in all of the city!

Producers, however, are problem solvers. And this man came up with a good one. Since he and his son—and an 85-year-old grandfather—all lived under one roof, it seemed logical that he could ask his son to read some of the highlights from the book in the evening hours.

Before they knew it, a ritual had begun. The son would read a portion of the book out loud every night to his father and his grandfather.

Well, it's not *Goodnight, Moon*, but I have to admit it touches my heart!

"*You can't eat your way out of pain.*"

—*The Daily Adele Dose*

• •

Date:

What I ate...for breakfast: _____
_____
_____

What I ate...for my morning hard-chew snacks: _____
_____

What I ate...for lunch: _____
_____
_____
_____

What I ate...for my afternoon soft chews: _____

What I ate...for dinner: _____
_____
_____
_____

How I felt: _____
_____
_____

How I kept moving: _____
_____
_____

What I drank: _____
_____

Did I eat an apple today? _____

TEST YOUR STRESS-FACTOR SAVVY

Okay, so we all know that stress is a fact of life. It's here and it's not going away. But we also know that we can do something about the way we handle stress. We can punch a pillow, punch a person, or punch the cellophane open on a bag of chips.

There are good ways and bad ways to handle stress—and the 5-Day Miracle Diet helps you find the good way that will have "miraculous" results!

See if you can discover the good from the bad in the stress-loaded statements below:

1. **Your significant other just slammed the door and walked out after a particularly draining fight. You:**
   (a) Cry hysterically as you pour an 8-ounce glass of whiskey.
   (b) Cry hysterically as you dig into the cold egg rolls and fried rice in the refrigerator.
   (c) Cry hysterically as you dial a close friend for comfort.

   Well, the crying is inevitable, and you could look at it as a catharsis. But only (c) calling a close friend will really help you through this difficult time. The other choices will ultimately make you feel worse.

2. **You visit your mother on Saturday, only to be told that you still have to lose weight and whatever did you do with your hair! You:**
   (a) Start to scream and, voice dripping with sarcasm, tell your mother that, in actuality, you're thinking of dying your hair purple and, combined with all your excess weight, maybe you'll be able to join the circus.
   (b) Whine and immediately walk over to the refrigerator to see what you can stuff into your mouth first.
   (c) Laugh it off and, shaking your head, say, "Mom, you're unbelievable. Come on, let's go to the movies."

   The right answer is (c). Get out of the house, which is a trigger. Make light of your mother's criticism. And go to a movie and enjoy the distraction. Please note: This response can require a combination of the 5-Day Miracle Diet and several years of therapy.

"The fathead only has as much power as you give it."
—*The Daily Adele Dose*

• •

Date: _____

What I ate...for breakfast: _____
_____
_____

What I ate...for my morning hard-chew snacks: _____
_____

What I ate...for lunch: _____
_____
_____
_____

What I ate...for my afternoon soft chews: _____

What I ate...for dinner: _____
_____
_____
_____

How I felt: _____
_____
_____

How I kept moving: _____
_____
_____

What I drank: _____
_____

Did I recognize and handle a fathead *issue today?* _____

AVOID FOOD CATASTROPHE: THINK OF YOURSELF!

Sara was one of those people who thought catastrophically when it came to the connection between food and the people in her life. If she refused the chocolate chip cookie her boss offered because she wasn't hungry, she'd be fired. If she told her boyfriend she just didn't feel like eating Chinese on Friday night, he'd walk out of her life for good. And if she told her best friend that she didn't want to eat her "I made this chocolate cake just for you" dessert because she'd rather save a "Food You Adore" item for a party the next night, her friend would never talk to her again.

Seeing these words in black-and-white makes them sound ridiculous—and they make Sara sound awfully neurotic. But there are many, many of us who intellectually understand that saying no is one's right but who, emotionally, break out in a cold sweat if they stand up to others. Sara was one of these people, which is why she was having trouble losing weight.

It wasn't just due to the *fathead* creed that she was eating her feelings; it was also the fact that she placed herself in tempting situations while feeling very vulnerable. Why eat that first chocolate chip cookie if she really didn't want it? Why go out to a Chinese restaurant, with all its fatty dishes, if she really didn't feel like eating steamed veggies and tofu? And why eat someone's dessert if she didn't even like chocolate! With sabotage like this in place, you're just setting yourself up to fail—and gain weight.

Once Sara's body got into good blood sugar on the 5-Day Miracle Diet, we began to work on this common—but dangerous—*fathead* issue. We rehearsed scenarios. Sara began to learn how to say no nicely, with a reassuring smile and a logical explanation.

I knew Sara "owned" the diet—and had reclaimed her life—when she came into my office on a Monday with an amazing story.

Sara's boss had asked her to finish an assignment on Friday night. But Sara had a dinner date with a friend. Like the Sara of yore, however, she said yes. She booted up her computer—and realized that the work would take her way past the time she was to meet her friend.

The *new* Sara turned the computer off. She got up from her chair and walked into her boss's office. She told her boss that she couldn't possibly finish the project that night. She took a deep breath, waiting for the tirade she knew would soon come. Wrong. Her boss merely smiled and said fine!

Sara was able to meet her friend on time for dinner. On Monday morning, she came in to the office a half hour earlier and finished the report.

Everyone was happy, especially Sara. She had learned a powerful lesson about herself.

"The world is a cornucopia of food choices. The fathead has only a limited menu."

—*The Daily Adele Dose*

• •

Date: _____

What I ate...for breakfast: _____

_____

_____

What I ate...for my morning hard-chew snacks: _____

_____

What I ate...for lunch: _____

_____

_____

_____

What I ate...for my afternoon soft chews: _____

What I ate...for dinner: _____

_____

_____

_____

How I felt: _____

_____

_____

How I kept moving: _____

_____

_____

What I drank: _____

_____

Did I scope the buffet table before filling my plate? _____

FILET MIGNON PIQUANT

A good quality cut of steak can be perfection by itself, but grilling and broiling and barbecuing can become boring. Add spark to your steak with this fabulous recipe, which adds a vegetable basil sauce that rivals its more fattening counterparts. Add a potato or rice, a salad with one of my dressings, and zucchini, and dinner is served!

What you'll need:

4 tablespoons extra-virgin olive oil
1 pound filet mignon, sliced into julienne strips
4 cups julienne-cut onions
4 cups sliced mushrooms
4 cups sliced bell peppers
4 cups chopped broccoli florets
2 sliced tomatoes
1 cup low-fat chicken stock
2 tablespoons chopped basil
   Salt and pepper to taste

What you'll do:

Heat 2 tablespoons of the oil in a large skillet until a drop of water sizzles in its center. Sauté all the vegetables, except the tomato, until golden. Remove vegetables and set aside.

Heat the same pan over high heat until very hot (about 1 minute). Add the remaining oil and the beef. Sauté the beef for 2 to 3 minutes. Add the tomato, chicken stock, basil, and salt and pepper to taste.

Add the vegetables and sauté until heated through.

Serves 4. Men: Add 1 ounce of protein to your salad. Don't forget to add the oil toward your daily allotment of fat.

MIRACLE DIET CHEF'S HINT: Feel free to exchange the filet mignon for a different meat. This dish is also delicious with chicken, pork, veal, or lamb.

"Did you ever think you'd have this much energy, this much drive, this much zest for life?"

—*The Daily Adele Dose*

• •

Date:

What I ate...for breakfast: _____
_____
_____

What I ate...for my morning hard-chew snacks: _____
_____

What I ate...for lunch: _____
_____
_____
_____

What I ate...for my afternoon soft chews: _____

What I ate...for dinner: _____
_____
_____
_____

How I felt: _____
_____
_____

How I kept moving: _____
_____
_____

What I drank: _____
_____

Did I eat the right amount of starches today? _____

Here's something one of my clients, an executive in a cosmetics firm, told me:

"When I get upset and I have some money, I go shopping. When I'm broke, I go eating."

THE THREE-STEP PLAN TO SUCCESS ON THE 5-DAY MIRACLE DIET

1. *Eat at specific times during the day.*

2. *Eat specific types of food.*

3. *Eat specific combinations and textures of food.*

> *"Doing something for you and you alone is not a bad thing."*
>
> —*The Daily Adele Dose*

• •

Date:

What I ate...for breakfast: _____

_____

_____

What I ate...for my morning hard-chew snacks: _____

_____

What I ate...for lunch: _____

_____

_____

_____

What I ate...for my afternoon soft chews: _____

What I ate...for dinner: _____

_____

_____

_____

How I felt: _____

_____

_____

How I kept moving: _____

_____

_____

What I drank: _____

_____

Did I "tie the bow" on my blood sugar with a hard chew at lunch today? _____

WEIGHTY ISSUES

Last week's weight: _____

Pounds lost: _____

New weight: _____

Don't forget those lost ounces and half pounds. They add up!

• •

When planning to eat in your office, don't order "in," order "out." Go for a short walk, clear your head, and choose exactly what you want from the corner coffee shop. You'll come back refreshed and ready to eat the right way!

• •

A WEEK'S "POCKETFUL OF MIRACLES"

*E*very week now, for several months, you've been thinking about the small—and big—miracles that have occurred in your life. Perhaps it's time to remember what the miracles are all about—before you start to take them for granted and they start to lose their power!

A 5-Day "Pocketful of Miracles" miracle is something that belongs to you and only you. It is an experience that has affected your life in a positive manner. It not only keeps motivation strong in the week ahead, but it helps you keep a weekly log of the exciting changes going in your body, your mind, and your soul. It shows you just how much your life is changing in wonderful ways!

Here's a miracle that spells it all out. It comes from one of my long-time clients:

•*Sure, there are little things that happen every day. True, it's amazing that I don't miss the morning bagel or the orange juice or the banana. But it's more than that. It's how I feel. I have so much energy that sometimes I don't even know myself! How did I ever exist before?*

Now it's your turn: _____

_____

_____

"If you control the way you eat in good blood sugar, you can control yourself in almost any situation."

—The Daily Adele Dose

• •

Date:

What I ate...for breakfast: _____
_____
_____

What I ate...for my morning hard-chew snacks: _____
_____

What I ate...for lunch: _____
_____
_____
_____

What I ate...for my afternoon soft chews: _____

What I ate...for dinner: _____
_____
_____
_____

How I felt: _____
_____
_____

How I kept moving: _____
_____
_____

What I drank: _____
_____

Did I eat lunch by 1:00 P.M.? _____

THE STORY OF THE WRITER AND THE
HÄAGEN-DAZS POP

Jake loved to cook. It was one of his passions (and, not incidentally, one of the reasons he had gained twenty pounds and needed to see me). By the time he was on the 5-Day Miracle Diet for two months, he'd already adapted many of his favorite recipes into low-fat, no-sugar versions. But every once in a while, he made his specialty: angel hair pasta and white clam sauce. Yum. He'd eat his portion as a "Food You Adore," and his company, well, they ate and ate and ate!

One night he'd invited his favorite aunt over for dinner. She was delighted, of course, but she had one request: the angel hair pasta dish. No problem. Jake was ready; he knew she adored it. And he planned to join her. Luckily, he hadn't yet had his "Food You Adore" for the week!

But he was in a quandary about dessert. He didn't want to bake anything that was too tempting, so he decided to buy some rich, chocolatey Häagen-Dazs pops. His aunt could eat one and take the rest home.

Unfortunately, Jake couldn't find good fresh clams for his recipe at any store. Disappointed, he tried to call his aunt and change their plans. But she wasn't home. Oh, well, he decided. They'd just go out to eat, his treat. They opted for an Italian restaurant, and Jake made the decision to stick to the 5-Day Miracle Diet. He'd have an ice-cream pop when they got back to the house.

After a satisfying meal of salad, grilled fish, and veggies, Jake felt fabulous. It was a lovely spring night, so he suggested they take a walk through the city streets. By the time he put his aunt in a taxi, he was ready to go to sleep. He decided to hold off once more on his "Food You Adore." The pops lay in the freezer. Quiet. Waiting.

The next morning, Jake opened the fridge to get his breakfast. Wanting ice for some water, he opened the freezer door. Ah! There they were, all wrapped up and no place to go. Jake quickly closed the door. He shrugged. After all, he was in GBS and he could have a pop as a "Food You Adore" any time he chose.

He chose that night, after work. He opened the freezer, took out a pop, and unwrapped it. Then he remembered: The next morning he had an important meeting. Jake knew it would take a day or two to get his blood sugar back in balance—and he didn't want to sit there yawning at the conference table because he was in low blood sugar! So Jake put the pop back. He'd save it for another time.

When Jake told this story to me during our regular session, I grinned from ear to ear. The whole process had come so naturally to him, he was now able to make real, conscious choices about his eating—and about his life.

> *"Take away the low-blood-sugar levels in your body and you will lose the physiological cravings for starches, sweets, alcohol, caffeine, and fats. And the 5-Day Miracle Diet makes it easy."*
>
> —*The Daily Adele Dose*

• •

Date:

What I ate...for breakfast: _____

_____

_____

What I ate...for my morning hard-chew snacks: _____

_____

What I ate...for lunch: _____

_____

_____

_____

What I ate...for my afternoon soft chews: _____

What I ate...for dinner: _____

_____

_____

_____

How I felt: _____

_____

_____

How I kept moving: _____

_____

_____

What I drank: _____

_____

Did I get off the bus one stop farther away from my office so I could walk? _____

Chicken Jardinière

This chicken recipe combines the cool pleasures and crunchiness of fresh garden vegetables with the tender warmth of sautéed chicken. Not only is it a beautiful dish to serve to those you love, but your taste buds will thank you, too!

What you'll need:
4–6 ounces skinless, boneless chicken breast
  4 cups chopped salad, made up of equal amounts of fresh, cleaned tomatoes, romaine lettuce, endive, arugula, and radicchio
    Tricolore Dressing (page 36), Charlotte Dressing (page 132), or Lemon-Tarragon Vinaigrette Dressing (page 216)
 ½ tablespoon oil, preferably canola or extra-virgin olive oil

What you'll do:
  Between two pieces of waxed paper, pound the chicken breast to double its size. Slice it into slivers or leave whole for one dinner serving.
  Mix the chopped salad together with one of the three dressings you'll find in this book. Store in the refrigerator for 5 minutes only.
  While the salad is chilling, heat the oil in a large frying pan. Add the chicken breast and sauté for 2 minutes on each side, or until light brown.
  Place the chicken on a plate and cover with the chilled salad.

Serves 1 (male-sized portion) or 2 (meals for women, lunch or dinner). Don't forget to add the oil and salad dressing toward your daily allotment of fat.

"*Food is love. How sad. How devious!*"

—*The Daily Adele Dose*

• •

Date:

What I ate...for breakfast: _____
_____
_____

What I ate...for my morning hard-chew snacks: _____
_____

What I ate...for lunch: _____
_____
_____
_____

What I ate...for my afternoon soft chews: _____

What I ate...for dinner: _____
_____
_____
_____

How I felt: _____
_____
_____

How I kept moving: _____
_____
_____

What I drank: _____
_____

Did I decide not *to eat something I love, because it wasn't the appropriate time or reason?* _____

IT MIGHT JUST BE FISH EGGS, BUT TO SOME IT'S THE FOOD OF THE GODS

Caviar is one of those precious foods we think of when we imagine heads of state entertaining in a large dining hall. The crystal is glistening. The caviar—black, shiny, perfectly whole, and firm—sits proudly in a bed of crushed ice. The toast points are perfectly cut in triangles for delicate caviar holders. And the chopped egg and onion await white-gloved fingertips for garnish.

In reality, anyone can buy caviar—and it even tastes great on a Ritz cracker! The best news about caviar is the fact that it isn't fattening. Although it does have more fat than other forms of fish, there's only about 70 calories per ounce, and it's all healthy. Plus it's fish—a protein that won't make you crave.

The only caviar that can call itself by its rightful name are those eggs that come from sturgeons. The three "kings" include:

✔ **Beluga**. The Main Man. A large, mild-tasting berry that is usually more gray than black.
✔ **Osetra**. This is an intense golden brown caviar.
✔ **Sevruga**. The tiniest eggs make up this "baby" caviar.

All three caviars are expensive and not for everyday consumption (unless, of course, you're related to an Arab sheik). You can do almost as well with lumpfish caviar (which is dyed red or black) and Keta, which comes from salmon and is naturally bright red. Both are delicious and about half the price of sturgeon roe.

There's only one problem with caviar: It's hard to eat just one spoonful. Save it for a "Food You Adore" and enjoy it with those triangular, perfectly toasted pieces of bread.

"When you're in good blood sugar, you just don't think about food. I know this. I experience this firsthand every day of my life. "

—The Daily Adele Dose

• •

Date:

What I ate...for breakfast: _____
_____
_____

What I ate...for my morning hard-chew snacks: _____
_____

What I ate...for lunch: _____
_____
_____
_____

What I ate...for my afternoon soft chews: _____

What I ate...for dinner: _____
_____
_____
_____

How I felt: _____
_____
_____

How I kept moving: _____
_____
_____

What I drank: _____
_____

Did I dream of food last night? _____

ONLY SKIN DEEP

We scrub it. We moisturize it. We loofah it. We shave it. And above all, we try to hide it—especially when we hate the way it looks. It's called skin and, despite all the brouhaha, it weighs only about six pounds!

"For several years, it bothered me that, as a healthy woman in my forties, I had so little energy. At the end of every day, I couldn't wait to get home and conk out. I was excited about my life, working on a new career, so I knew I wasn't bored or depressed. What could be wrong? The 5-Day Miracle Diet has turned all that around. I am working two demanding jobs, taking classes three nights a week, and juggling other activities. I know the energy to do all that comes from your diet, Adele. Thank you!"

—A professor who began the 5-Day Miracle Diet four months ago

"We can't change stress but we can change the way we handle it."

—*The Daily Adele Dose*

• •

Date:

What I ate...for breakfast: _____
_____
_____

What I ate...for my morning hard-chew snacks: _____
_____

What I ate...for lunch: _____
_____
_____
_____

What I ate...for my afternoon soft chews: _____

What I ate...for dinner: _____
_____
_____
_____

How I felt: _____
_____
_____

How I kept moving: _____
_____
_____

What I drank: _____
_____

Did I try creative visualization or imagery to reduce my stress?
_____

Lemon-Tarragon Vinaigrette Dressing

This flavorful dressing is ideal for garden salads or fresh crudités and as a marinade for chicken and fish. It has a zesty tang that makes everything taste delicious!

What you'll need:

¼ cup tarragon vinegar
¼ cup fresh lemon juice
¼ cup water
2 tablespoons extra-virgin olive oil
1 tablespoon Dijon mustard
  Pinch of oregano, chopped or dried
  Salt and pepper to taste

What you'll do:

Mix all the ingredients in a bowl, using a whisk. Store in a covered container in the refrigerator. Shake before using.

Serves 4. Don't forget to add the oil to your daily fat allotment.

"Learn to distract yourself when food starts saying hello."

—*The Daily Adele Dose*

• •

Date:

What I ate...for breakfast: _____
_____
_____

What I ate...for my morning hard-chew snacks: _____
_____

What I ate...for lunch: _____
_____
_____
_____

What I ate...for my afternoon soft chews: _____

What I ate...for dinner: _____
_____
_____
_____

How I felt: _____
_____
_____

How I kept moving: _____
_____
_____

What I drank: _____
_____

Did I go out for a walk today? _____

THE FAMILY DINNER AND DESSERT

Some people remember their years growing up with flashes of Christmas trees, snow-covered trails, or summers canoeing by the lake. They remember the laughter, the camaraderie, the daring. Others remember their youth through food: the chicken Mother used to make, the ices sold on the corner, the one-penny candy hoarded in sticky pockets. Still others remember food as a catalyst, a learned response, that made for other memories, funny now but completely serious then.

Take Kathy, a medical researcher who'd been in to see me for three months now. She'd already lost seventeen pounds on the 5-Day Miracle Diet and she was beginning to think about her food issues, how her entire life had revolved around food and gaining weight.

Kathy hated liver with a passion. A popular dish not so long ago, liver was considered healthy, chock-full of iron. Today, we know it's also chock-full of cholesterol and other toxins, but back then it was almost required eating once a week, sautéed in oil and served with smothered onions.

Whenever Kathy got home from school and saw a familiar green-and-brown striped bakery box tied with string, she never had to ask "What's for dinner?" It would be liver. Way before she'd start cooking, her mother would have gone to the bakery and picked up the richest and most beautifully iced cupcakes. It was Kathy's reward for eating her liver!

Until Kathy recognized her **Bad Food/Good Food** *fathead* during several months of discussion in my office, she'd subconsciously reward herself with a thickly iced cupcake whenever she had to do something particularly unpleasant.

Today she no longer rewards herself with food. But she still won't go near liver.

"Putting yourself first. What a concept! What a joy!"
—*The Daily Adele Dose*

• •

Date:

What I ate…for breakfast: _____
_____
_____

What I ate…for my morning hard-chew snacks: _____
_____

What I ate…for lunch: _____
_____
_____
_____

What I ate…for my afternoon soft chews: _____

What I ate…for dinner: _____
_____
_____
_____

How I felt: _____
_____
_____

How I kept moving: _____
_____
_____

What I drank: _____
_____

Did I stand up for myself at work today? _____

WEIGHTY ISSUES

Last week's weight: _____

Pounds lost: _____

New weight: _____

*Don't forget those lost ounces and half
pounds. They add up!*

• •

*Remember, menus aren't written in stone. Chefs can adapt
and modify dishes according to your needs—and they can
still be delicious. Restaurants have lots of foods and spices
in their kitchens, and chefs like to be creative!*

• •

A WEEK'S "POCKETFUL OF MIRACLES"

A miracle can take many guises. It can be as complicated as healing
the sick or getting pregnant after years and years of trying. It can be as
wonderful as winning the lottery or making a child smile.

Some miracles are quieter than others. They are the achievements
that we alone have accomplished—and that we alone can understand
and feel the joy of.

These are the miracles I am talking about in your 5-Day Miracle Diet
journey. Maybe you signed up for an exercise class. Or maybe you
threw the rest of your child's Happy Meal away instead of nibbling at
the fried stuff—and smiled all the way home.

Here's a miracle from a man who'd written me after reading my
book:

•*A good friend brought over a box of chocolates last night. We each ate
only one and happily gave the rest to a neighbor.*

Now it's your turn: _____

_____

_____

"Habit is one of the most potent tools our fathead sabo-teurs have. The one defense? Break the link and change the habit!"

—*The Daily Adele Dose*

• •

Date:

What I ate...for breakfast: _____

_____

_____

What I ate...for my morning hard-chew snacks: _____

_____

What I ate...for lunch: _____

_____

_____

_____

What I ate...for my afternoon soft chews: _____

What I ate...for dinner: _____

_____

_____

_____

How I felt: _____

_____

_____

How I kept moving: _____

_____

_____

What I drank: _____

_____

Did I try eating dinner in another room, just to change the routine?

_____

AN EMBARRASSING MOMENT

Picture this scenario. You've been invited to a good friend's house for dinner. Everyone knows you're on the 5-Day Miracle Diet because you've had to tell them where you've gotten this boundless energy and new lease on life.

So far so good. But when you get to the house, you find out it's a surprise party—for you. To celebrate your fortieth birthday.

Of course, you are touched. You see all your friends' smiling faces; you are with people you love and who love you.

There's just one glitch: You hadn't planned on making this a "Food You Adore" night and you notice this chocolate sheet cake in the middle of a fabulous buffet. The cake says "Happy Birthday!" How can you refuse?

It might not be a birthday party. It might just be a night out at a friend's apartment. Or a holiday meal at your grandmother's house. Whatever it is, here are some hints to keep you in good blood sugar without alienating your family and friends. And oh, yes, have a good time, too!

- *Treat your hard chews like first-aid kits.* Take a plastic bag of veggies wherever you go, especially when you're going to a friend's house for dinner. Excuse yourself for a moment. Go down the hall and gobble one of the carrots. Your blood chemistry will be stable and you'll be more inclined to stick with your diet plan.
- *People are busy talking at parties.* If you move the fattening potatoes or cheese sauces to the side, no one will notice—especially if you bring your own plate (piled underneath two others) into the kitchen to help out!
- *Many people are watching their fat intake today.* Most probably, you'll find platters of crudités and shrimp on ice as readily as you would the six-foot subs. And speaking of subs, you can carefully eat a slice of tomato, some onion, and a bit of lettuce from the sandwich without taking a bite of bread or fattening deli meat!
- *If you don't eat sheet cake, you can still appreciate it—without hurting your friend's feelings.* Blow out your candles. Exclaim how beautiful the cake looks. Cut slices for everyone except yourself. No one will notice if you have a cup in hand.
- *If perchance your friend does notice you haven't touched her cake, give her a great big hug.* Tell her how touched and happy you are with the entire affair. She made such a fabulous meal that you're not hungry right now. Maybe later. Tell her you love her—and mean it!
- *If your friend suggests you take a piece home, say "fine."* Simply toss it or give it away when you leave her home.
- *Above all, enjoy your party.* You don't turn forty every day! Make the choices *you* want.

"The miracle comes when you change something for the better in your life!"

—*The Daily Adele Dose*

• •

Date:

What I ate...for breakfast: _____

_____

_____

What I ate...for my morning hard-chew snacks: _____

_____

What I ate...for lunch: _____

_____

_____

_____

What I ate...for my afternoon soft chews: _____

What I ate...for dinner: _____

_____

_____

_____

How I felt: _____

_____

_____

How I kept moving: _____

_____

_____

What I drank: _____

_____

Did I stop using words like good *and* bad *when describing my diet?*

_____

MÉLANGE OF FRUITS WITH BERRY DIP

The afternoon is time for maintenance.
Your blood sugar is balanced, and all
you have to do is keep it that way.
Soft-chew fruits are perfect for that
vitalized, energized balance. This exquisite fruit platter is perfect for company during teatime or anytime you want to make a leisurely afternoon special.

What you'll need:

For fruit platter:

- 2 apricots, pitted
- 2 kiwis, peeled
- 2 peaches, pitted
- ½ cup fresh raspberries
- 1 orange, shell only, for garnish

For dip:

- ½ pint fresh raspberries
- ½ pint fresh blackberries
- 8 medium strawberries, hulled
- ½ pint fresh blueberries

What you'll do:

Cut apricots, kiwis, and peaches into 8 slices each. Arrange all the fruit on a dish surrounding the hollow orange shell.

Purée dip ingredients for 2 minutes in a blender or food processor. Strain the purée through a very fine mesh strainer, removing seeds.

Pour the dip into the orange shell to serve.

Serves 10 (or 5 used as a double fruit allotment). Since the fruits in this recipe are soft chews, they can be used in the afternoon or as an occasional dessert after dinner.

"Vegetables scrub out your cells. Fruit eliminates the 'scrub out' from your body. Combine this with eight or more glasses of water a day, and you have a smooth movement through your intestines—which makes your body metabolically clean, healthy, and less likely to retain water!"

—*The Daily Adele Dose*

• •

Date:

What I ate...for breakfast: _____

_____

_____

What I ate...for my morning hard-chew snacks: _____

_____

What I ate...for lunch: _____

_____

_____

_____

What I ate...for my afternoon soft chews: _____

What I ate...for dinner: _____

_____

_____

_____

How I felt: _____

_____

_____

How I kept moving: _____

_____

_____

What I drank: _____

_____

Did I make sure my hard-chew pear was not too ripe?_____

Maybe It's the Microwave

Popcorn is one of the most "pop"-ular snack foods around today. In fact, the American Popcorn Institute has found that we eat close to 8 billion quarts of popcorn every year! But only about 10 percent of that corn is found in movie theaters. Most of us prefer to eat our popcorn behind closed doors, at home.

Now aren't you glad it's a "Food You Adore," allowed on the 5-Day Miracle Diet!

EAT HEARTY, FOR TOMORROW YOU DIET

Ancient Egyptian priests knew how to throw a party. Amidst the platters of fruits, vegetables, and beans was a mummy. Yes, a mummy. Although it's not clear if it had the place of honor, the mummy sat during all the festivities to remind everyone that even while they were enjoying a fabulous feast, death was present. Talk about hard chews!

> *"Like the classic childhood tale, tell yourself, 'I know I can!' Because you can!"*
>
> *—The Daily Adele Dose*

• •

Date:

What I ate...for breakfast: _____

_____

_____

What I ate...for my morning hard-chew snacks: _____

_____

What I ate...for lunch: _____

_____

_____

_____

What I ate...for my afternoon soft chews: _____

What I ate...for dinner: _____

_____

_____

_____

How I felt: _____

_____

_____

How I kept moving: _____

_____

_____

What I drank: _____

_____

Did I use my chopsticks to wipe the excess sauce off my Chinese food today? _____

SPORT CHECK

Here's a brief listing of some activities that we love to do—and how good they are for us:

- Racquetball, basketball, cross-country skiing, soccer, aerobic walking, and handball are the best exercises for cardiovascular fitness and burning calories.

- Next on the list are aerobics, crew, mountain hiking, golf, canoeing, fencing, tennis, and ice and in-line skating.

- Down on the bottom (but still good for you!) are horseback riding, swimming, downhill skiing, bowling, archery, sailing, and karate.

> *"Seeing is believing. Look in the mirror and see the powerful, healthy new you!"*
>
> *—The Daily Adele Dose*

• •

Date: _____

What I ate...for breakfast: _____
_____
_____

What I ate...for my morning hard-chew snacks: _____
_____

What I ate...for lunch: _____
_____
_____
_____

What I ate...for my afternoon soft chews: _____

What I ate...for dinner: _____
_____
_____
_____

How I felt: _____
_____
_____

How I kept moving: _____
_____
_____

What I drank: _____
_____

Did I look at myself in the mirror fully clothed? _____

LIFE AFTER PASTA

I know. It's hard to believe that you can live, let alone happily live, without pasta, at least most of the time. But you can. I *stripped the carbs* a long time ago, and it's been great ever since. I have my pasta once in a while, but it's not a foodfest craving. I'm in control, and I occasionally choose pasta as my "Food I Adore." I promise: The cravings will decrease once you, too, spend five days *stripping the carbs*.

Here are some hints to help you adjust to a "world without bread" while you're waiting for the cravings to crawl away:

✔ Stay in good blood sugar. You're more sensitive to blood-sugar fluctuations than non–carbohydrate addicts, and if you're not in good blood sugar, it's like a double whammy.
✔ Get the bread basket away—fast.
✔ Immediately order a salad in a restaurant. This way you can crunch away with the bread eaters at the table.
✔ Stay away from the supermarket aisles that are labeled spaghetti, cereal, and tropical produce.
✔ Discover the delicious joys of beans, exotic rice, and lentils. No, they're not pasta, but sometimes they're even better!
✔ Bring your veggies and water on the plane with you. Tell your flight attendant to take away any bread, rolls, or starchy desserts that are sitting on your food tray.
✔ Eat seconds of veggies and protein when you dine at a friend's house. They will be so happy about your "May I have some more, please?" they won't even notice that you're not eating any starch.

"Do you feel it? You're getting the rhythm. You're feeling lighter. Your feet are positively ten feet off the ground! It's called good blood sugar!"

—*The Daily Adele Dose*

• •

Date:

What I ate...for breakfast: _____
_____
_____

What I ate...for my morning hard-chew snacks: _____
_____

What I ate...for lunch: _____
_____
_____
_____

What I ate...for my afternoon soft chews: _____

What I ate...for dinner: _____
_____
_____
_____

How I felt: _____
_____
_____

How I kept moving: _____
_____
_____

What I drank: _____
_____

*Did I turn on some music today and just start dancing for ten minutes or so?*_____

SHRIMP AND ARUGULA LINGUINE

Pasta lovers everywhere—and that always includes me!—will enjoy this delicious dish. As long as you are not a carbohydrate addict, you can enjoy this wonderful repast on the 5-Day Miracle Diet at dinner every other day. Add a salad with one of my dressings and you have one of the most delicious, nutritious, and simple meals I've ever had the pleasure to make and eat! *Mangia!*

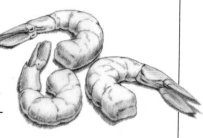

What you'll need:

- 2 tablespoons extra-virgin olive oil
- 8 cloves garlic, sliced
- 24 large shrimp
- 8 ounces linguine
- ¼ cup linguine cooking water
- 2 bunches arugula, rinsed and coarsely chopped
- 8 ripe plum (Roma) tomatoes, cut into chunks
  Basil to taste
  Salt and pepper to taste

What you'll do:

Heat the oil in a large skillet and sauté the garlic until golden. Add the shrimp and sauté for 2 minutes.

Cook the linguine in salted water for 5 minutes. Drain, saving ¼ cup of the cooking water. Set aside.

Add tomatoes, arugula, and basil, salt and pepper to taste, and the linguine water to the mixture in the skillet. Bring to a boil.

Add the linguine and continue boiling for 1 minute.

Serves 4 (male-sized portions). Note that 1 cup of pasta equals two servings of starch. Women should put approximately ¼ cup of the dish in a plastic container and eat it as an accompaniment for dinner in two nights.

"Don't live for your 'Foods You Adore.' Let them come, let them be relished, but don't deprive yourself the rest of the week in anticipation! There are a lot more everyday Miracle Diet days to experience!"

—The Daily Adele Dose

• •

Date:

What I ate...for breakfast: _____
_____
_____

What I ate...for my morning hard-chew snacks: _____
_____

What I ate...for lunch: _____
_____
_____
_____

What I ate...for my afternoon soft chews: _____

What I ate...for dinner: _____
_____
_____
_____

How I felt: _____
_____
_____

How I kept moving: _____
_____
_____

What I drank: _____
_____

Did I plan my "Food You Adore" while in good blood sugar?
_____

Yet another month has gone by and the weight is coming off—or is it? Now's the time to take a good, hard look at what you've been doing and see if you've been succeeding.

Success takes many forms. Yours might show in a steady weight loss. On the other hand, I have many clients who have found that weight is much less important now that they feel confident, strong, and capable. Success can even be something as "minor" as cutting back on caffeine, limiting red meat to once or twice a month, or using the stairs instead of the elevator.

The important concept to remember this month is the many faces of success. Evaluate yourself both in the bigger picture and on the small screen.

By examining your entire lifestyle, you'll find success in some surprising places—and it will keep you going just when you've decided to quit.

Remember, the more months you are on the 5-Day Miracle Diet, the more you follow the basic rules and face your *fathead* issues, the more you will "own" the diet. And once you own it, no one, I repeat, no one, can ever take it away from you again.

I call this empowerment at its finest.

Good luck next month!

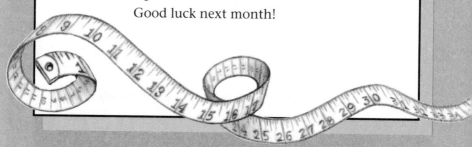

Inch-by-Inch

Bust/chest: _____   Upper arms: _____

Wrists: _____   Waist: _____

Abdomen: _____   Hips and buttocks: _____

IN A WORD...

Sum up your monthly experience in one or two words. Use it as your "mantra" in the month to come. It's easy now that you've made the 5-Day Miracle Diet yours to keep! Here's one of my favorites:

Why didn't I do this sooner!

What's your good word?

_____

Shout it out. You should feel proud!

You can get your exercise any time and anywhere. Do some "arm curls" with two bottles of water from the fridge. Roll two 8-ounce cans under your bare feet for leg stretches. Stretch your arms up, holding your stomach in, when you change a lightbulb!

How important is food to you, really?

If you were stranded, which would you choose: chocolate cake or good company? Kind of puts those seductive foods into perspective!

WEIGHTY ISSUES

Last week's weight: _____

Pounds lost: _____

New weight: _____

*Don't forget those lost ounces and half
pounds. They add up!*

• •

*Remember that to live a good, exciting life you must never stop
learning—about people, about the world around you, and, yes,
about food. You can always learn to eat better, smarter, and
healthier throughout your life.*

• •

A WEEK'S "POCKETFUL OF MIRACLES"

*I*t's amazing. Every letter I receive, every phone call I get, there's a
person on the other end thanking me for changing his or her life.

I am eternally grateful and moved that I have been able to help
people, but as I say to them, and I'll say to you, "It's not me. It's you.
You're the miracle maker."

I can show you the way. I can describe the 5-Day Miracle Diet
basics. I can discuss how to pinpoint your *fathead* issues. But it's you
who must make the commitment. I cannot take credit for your daily
triumphs. But I can be happy for you. Very, very happy.

And nothing pleases me more than hearing about those daily triumphs, those miracles that all of you out there make happen. This
week, think about the miracles that have made you a "miracle maker."
Here's one I'm particularly fond of:

•*This week, after months on your diet, I didn't even think about dieting or
losing weight. I just went about my business. And then it struck me: I was
relaxed! What an amazing feeling.*

Now it's your turn: _____

_____

_____

"Make the diet work for you when you're in the morning rush. Think about what you'll eat for breakfast while you're planning what to wear!"

—*The Daily Adele Dose*

• •

Date:

What I ate...for breakfast: _____
_____
_____

What I ate...for my morning hard-chew snacks: _____

What I ate...for lunch: _____
_____
_____
_____

What I ate...for my afternoon soft chews: _____

What I ate...for dinner: _____
_____
_____
_____

How I felt: _____
_____
_____

How I kept moving: _____
_____
_____

What I drank: _____
_____

Did I do my basic weekly shopping? _____

ZUCCHINI ROMA

One of my personal quests is to find new, exciting ways to serve vegetables—a staple of the 5-Day Miracle Diet. Using vitamin-rich zucchini, this marvelous side dish has a hint of basil and chives in every bite. A festive dish to get rid of the vegetable blahs!

What you'll need:

- 8 6-inch-long zucchini
- 2 tablespoons extra-virgin olive oil
- 3 cups chopped scallions
- 3 cups chopped celery, white stalks only
- 3 cups chopped onions
- ½ chopped red bell pepper

- 4 mushroom caps, cleaned and chopped
- 3 cups chopped fresh spinach
- 12 chopped basil leaves
- 2 tablespoons chopped chives
- 1 tablespoon beaten egg whites
- 2 sliced plum (Roma) tomatoes
- Salt and pepper to taste

What you'll do:

To prepare zucchini for stuffing:

Preheat the oven to 350° F. Scrub the zucchini with a vegetable brush, removing skin. Slice them in half lengthwise. Remove the soft meat, leaving the shell. Place the zucchini shells in a shallow baking pan. Sprinkle with salt and pepper. Bake for 25 minutes. (Instead of baking, you can also boil the zucchini for 2 minutes in boiling, lightly salted water.)

To make stuffing:

Heat a 4-quart saucepan over high heat until a drop of water sizzles in its center. Add the oil, scallions, celery, onions, peppers, and mushrooms. Turn the heat to medium-low and simmer for 5 minutes, stirring occasionally.

Remove the saucepan from the heat and add the spinach, basil, chives, and egg whites and salt and pepper to taste.

Fill the zucchini halves with stuffing and bake for 7 minutes.

While the zucchini is cooking:

Place the tomato halves under the broiler (with oven still on 400° F). Serve zucchini and tomatoes together.

Serves 4 (2 zucchini each). Don't forget to add the oil toward your daily allotment of fat.

"Got the blues? Try singing. Food won't solve it!"

—*The Daily Adele Dose*

• •

Date:

What I ate...for breakfast: _____

_____

_____

What I ate...for my morning hard-chew snacks: _____

_____

What I ate...for lunch: _____

_____

_____

_____

What I ate...for my afternoon soft chews: _____

What I ate...for dinner: _____

_____

_____

_____

How I felt: _____

_____

_____

How I kept moving: _____

_____

_____

What I drank: _____

_____

Am I making sure I weigh myself only once a week? _____

EMPOWERMENT IS
AS EMPOWERMENT DOES

It's a simple statement but it's amazingly true. People who control their blood sugar become more powerful in every aspect of their lives.

I know. I've seen it happen to thousands of clients and readers who have embraced the 5-Day Miracle Diet.

What happens is this:

1. The good blood sugar makes people feel physically better and mentally alert.

2. This physical strength translates into a stronger sense of self, a confidence that simply wasn't there before.

3. This confidence strengthens resolve and enables people to say:

> "I have to eat dinner now, not later."
>
> "Please take this back to the kitchen. I asked for a salad with dressing on the side."
>
> "This dessert looks fabulous, but I am so stuffed from the delicious dinner you made. Maybe later."
>
> "No, thank you. I'll have a sparkling water instead."

4. When you learn to say these things, head high, you develop a strong sense of self, a positive, healthy sense of yourself that cannot be taken away by anybody—and which will flow into every aspect of your life!

"Good blood sugar is a friend for life!"

—The Daily Adele Dose

• •

Date:

What I ate...for breakfast: _____
_____
_____

What I ate...for my morning hard-chew snacks: _____
_____

What I ate...for lunch: _____
_____
_____
_____

What I ate...for my afternoon soft chews: _____

What I ate...for dinner:_____
_____
_____
_____

How I felt: _____
_____
_____

How I kept moving: _____
_____
_____

What I drank: _____
_____

Did I make sure I chose one or two "Foods You Adore" every week?
_____

TEST YOUR LUNCH-WITH-YOUR-BOSS SAVVY

Does the idea of breaking bread with your boss make you break out in a cold sweat? Are you afraid you'll forget which fork to use when he breaks the news—let along remember to "tie the bow" on your good blood sugar? Take a look at these situations and see if you "own" the 5-Day Miracle Diet enough to conquer even the *fathead*'s *fathead*: The Boss.

1. Your boss orders a double Scotch on the rocks. You:
(a) Tell him you're on a diet and grimace as you take a sip of luke-warm table water.
(b) Clearly and simply order a San Pellegrino and lime. If he protests, you simply smile and assure him that you are having a great time—and that you might join him in a drink later.
(c) Decide to do him one better and order a tequila, a lemon, and a shaker of salt.

The correct answer is (b). You don't have to explain anything. You can do as you want in a confident, poised manner.

2. You're sitting at a table looking at a menu that has nothing but pasta. You:
(a) Ask your waiter if it is possible to simply order a side salad with some cheese or chicken—and dressing on the side.
(b) Decide to order the special pasta with sausage, cheese, and olive oil. Hey, you're probably going to get fired anyway!
(c) Sit there and eat nothing, watching your boss consume a massive bowl of pasta.

The correct answer is (a). There's always a solution if you want to find it!

3. Your boss orders coffee and is about to tell you his news. But first he asks if you want dessert. You:
(a) Accidentally spill your water glass on your clean plate. You say excuse me while your stomach gurgles with hunger.
(b) Decide the worst and order the worst: a tiramisu that's so rich even you can't eat more than two bites.
(c) Shake your head no and order a decaf espresso. You take a breath and await the news: You've received a promotion! *Congratulations!*

The correct answer is (c). Not because it has a happy ending, but because no matter what the news was, you stayed in good blood sugar. You decided to take control of your life. You chose empowerment over victimization.

"Here's to your strong, marvelous, energetic new life!"
—*The Daily Adele Dose*

• •

Date:

What I ate...for breakfast: _____
_____

What I ate...for my morning hard-chew snacks: _____
_____

What I ate...for lunch: _____
_____
_____
_____

What I ate...for my afternoon soft chews: _____

What I ate...for dinner: _____
_____
_____
_____

How I felt: _____
_____
_____

How I kept moving: _____
_____
_____

What I drank: _____
_____

Did I walk down the hall a little taller today? _____

!!!SHOPPING MANIA!!!

Rule number one: If you don't make food shopping easy and convenient, you won't go the whole "five" yards. Shopping, cooking, and preparing must all be handy, efficient, and simple so you can succeed.

Stop number one? The supermarket. It's where the diet begins every week.

Here are a few shopping tips to facilitate your program and make trips to the supermarket an exercise in empowerment:

✔ Okay, we all know this one: Don't go to the supermarket hungry or in a craving mode. You'll end up buying that cute little mousse cake or a snack you can't pronounce or a pasta made from beets.

✔ Purchase major items only once a week. Friday nights are especially good. For some reason, most stores are empty. (Has *Friends* moved to Friday nights?)

✔ Major items include veggies, fruit, meats, no-fat cheeses, chicken, breads and rice, couscous, and one box of pasta.

✔ Do not, I repeat, do not go to the supermarket if you are feeling vulnerable, wired, or sad. The old *fathead* will rear its head and make you buy those seductive, dangerous items even though your body's in good blood sugar!

✔ Plan on one fast stop during the week, at either a convenience store or a greengrocer. Why? For perishables such as salads, skim milk for cereal, and any item you've run out of and need to keep that fabulous energy going on the 5-Day Miracle Diet!

"My program offers you three things: a reason, a choice, and freedom from food."

—The Daily Adele Dose

● ●

Date:

What I ate...for breakfast: _____

_____

_____

What I ate...for my morning hard-chew snacks: _____

_____

What I ate...for lunch: _____

_____

_____

_____

What I ate...for my afternoon soft chews: _____

What I ate...for dinner: _____

_____

_____

_____

How I felt: _____

_____

_____

How I kept moving: _____

_____

_____

What I drank: _____

_____

Did I eat berries after dinner instead of dessert? _____

A COFFEE-SHOP CHEW

Not every day brings you to the chic French restaurant everyone's talking about. Sometimes you don't have time for anything more than a coffee-shop lunch. Maybe you've done some errands and you don't feel like going back to the office yet. Maybe you don't want to eat lunch at your desk. Maybe you want an inexpensive, fast lunch.

Whatever the reason, coffee shops can be convenient places to stop for a meal. But they can also be dens of temptation. Burger platters. Cole slaw. Grilled cheese sandwiches. Revolving platters spinning with desserts. Help!

There's no reason why you can't march into a coffee shop on the 5-Day Miracle Diet. After all, the diet is designed to fit into your life—not the other way around. Here are some suggestions:

- ✓ Order sliced turkey, tomato and lettuce, and a side salad with oil and vinegar on the side. Opt for an optional slice of rye bread or a small roll.
- ✓ Chef salads are a good choice. Ask for yours made only with turkey—and don't eat it all! (Leave about a quarter of the turkey on the bottom with the soggy lettuce.)
- ✓ Have a souvlaki sandwich, but order yours made without fat. You'll receive a delicious pita filled with the right allotment of lamb, plus onions and tomatoes.
- ✓ Stay away from the pickles. They are very high in salt.
- ✓ Order scrambled eggs and a side salad, or an egg-white omelet made with veggies. Tell the waiter to hold the fat. They won't, but at least they'll know you're watching!

Most likely, you won't use your "Food You Adore" in a coffee shop. But just in case the temptation's in place, here are some suggestions for yummy "Extras":

- ✓ A tunafish sandwich on rye with lettuce and tomato
- ✓ That ubiquitous grilled cheese sandwich
- ✓ A burger platter with some of the fixings
- ✓ Homemade chicken soup and crackers

"Planning ahead doesn't take any complicated lists. It means making your veggies the night before, shopping for food once a week, and—for the fun part—deciding what 'Food You Adore' you'll decide to eat in the next seven days!"

—*The Daily Adele Dose*

· ·

Date:

What I ate...for breakfast: _____

_____

_____

What I ate...for my morning hard-chew snacks: _____

_____

What I ate...for lunch: _____

_____

_____

_____

What I ate...for my afternoon soft chews: _____

What I ate...for dinner: _____

_____

_____

_____

How I felt: _____

_____

_____

How I kept moving: _____

_____

_____

What I drank: _____

_____

Did I add lemon to my water for variety? _____

Is There Life After Relapse? No Problem!

A relapse is a learning experience. Everyone, at some time or another, has "relapsed." In fact, I don't even like to use the word. After all, you can't relapse from something you own!

But you can overindulge on occasion without it becoming a way of life. When you've eaten and drunk at a New Year's Eve bash, for example, there's always the next day. Before the big game, take a jog around the block. Put on some music and dance. Or if a hangover makes nothing possible except, perhaps, death, simply start fresh: Eat your 5-Day Miracle Diet breakfast within a half hour of waking up and get on with your day.

Expect some cravings during the next few days as your body readjusts. But they will pass. And you will soon be back on track!

"The 5-Day Miracle Diet is more than 'just a diet plan.' It becomes an act of love—self-love. It becomes an act of affirmation—for who you are and the respect you deserve."

—*The Daily Adele Dose*

• •

Date:

What I ate...for breakfast: _____
_____
_____

What I ate...for my morning hard-chew snacks: _____
_____

What I ate...for lunch: _____
_____
_____
_____

What I ate...for my afternoon soft chews: _____

What I ate...for dinner: _____
_____
_____
_____

How I felt: _____
_____
_____

How I kept moving: _____
_____
_____

What I drank: _____
_____

Did I try a new lipstick or a new aftershave today? _____

WEEKLY ASSESSMENT

WEIGHTY ISSUES

Last week's weight: _____

Pounds lost: _____

New weight: _____

Don't forget those lost ounces and half pounds. They add up!

• •

Seconds? Nothing tastes as good as the "first time." Savor the memory and let others be "seconds-best"!

• •

A WEEK'S "POCKETFUL OF MIRACLES"

*S*ometimes miracles are hard to find, especially if you're not looking for them. If you're feeling overly stressed or anxious, if you have had a disappointment in your work or personal life, you're not going to have as positive an outlook as you could.

The answer? Take a few moments while you read this sidebar and think about the past week. Remember the past few days at the office. Did you stand up for yourself, rather than feed your feelings? Did you bypass a food temptation?

And at home. Did you discover that a food craving was really an expression of anger, a *fathead*'s way to cope? After you put the kids to sleep, did you take a long, hot shower or a luxurious bath instead of sprawling out in front of the tube as you usually do?

Think about even the smallest "miracle" that might have occurred in your life. Here's a good one to fit this mood:

•*I had a horrible week, but I actually stayed on the 5-Day Miracle Diet. I didn't "give in to my* fathead*" as I usually would!*

Now it's your turn: _____

_____

_____

"People from all walks of life have come over to me during my travels and said 'You saved my life.' I say, 'No, you saved your life!'"

—*The Daily Adele Dose*

• •

Date:

What I ate...for breakfast: _____
_____
_____

What I ate...for my morning hard-chew snacks: _____
_____

What I ate...for lunch: _____
_____
_____
_____

What I ate...for my afternoon soft chews: _____

What I ate...for dinner: _____
_____
_____
_____

How I felt: _____
_____
_____

How I kept moving: _____
_____
_____

What I drank: _____
_____

Did I say thank you today when someone complimented me?
_____

TEST YOUR TRAVELING SAVVY

You're on a business trip, the kind of stress-producing roller-coaster ride that is ready to make you forget the 5-Day Miracle Diet for good. Let's see how well you will cope the next time you find yourself in a hotel room with a laptop, a wrinkled suit, and a project that's due the next morning...no matter what:

1. The room service menu is extensive. You have to work well into the night, so you decide to order:

(a) The hamburger deluxe, a piece of apple pie, and some cheese and crackers for later. After all, you feel deprived enough.
(b) A plate of crudités, heavy on the carrots and other hard chews. If you have to stay up late, you might as well have vigor and focus.
(c) A Diet Coke. You'll show "them." You'll not only stay up late, but you'll make it a real sacrifice!

This one's easy: It's (b). If you have to stay up all night, you might as well be smart about it. A carrot can go much further than a soggy, sluggish, cold piece of pie!

2. At breakfast the next morning, you remember the days before the 5-Day Miracle Diet when "brunch" was a once-a-week habit. You:

(a) Decide to order the whole deluxe breakfast package. After all, you were up all night. You deserve it!
(b) Don't even look at the menu. You know what breakfast fare looks like. Instead, you ask the waiter for a box of Wheat Chex, skim milk, and a big glass of ice-cold water.
(c) Purchase the newspaper and go back upstairs—where you've put your hard chews, low-fat cheese, and whole-grain bread in the hotel fridge.

The correct answer is (c), because it shows you are prepared—not only for your meeting, but for the 5-Day Miracle Diet as well! Although (b) is a correct breakfast, it will leave you empty if you don't have your hard chews to back it up an hour later. And besides, there's a whiff of deprivation in the dining room air. Better to go upstairs in your vulnerable state and not even face the pancakes at the next table!

3. In your carry-on suitcase, next to your portable hair dryer and your extra underwear, you packed:

(a) A Snickers bar
(b) Cut-up carrots, string beans, and cauliflower in little plastic bags
(c) A vial of vodka

This one is so easy, it shouldn't even be here! The answer is (b). Call it a reminder: Always pack your hard chews when you travel—just in case of emergency!

"Fight the physiological force that makes you crave. Get in good blood sugar today!"

—*The Daily Adele Dose*

• •

Date:

What I ate...for breakfast: _____

_____

What I ate...for my morning hard-chew snacks: _____

_____

What I ate...for lunch: _____

_____

_____

What I ate...for my afternoon soft chews: _____

What I ate...for dinner: _____

_____

_____

How I felt: _____

_____

How I kept moving: _____

_____

What I drank: _____

_____

Did I eat dinner at an appropriate time? _____

CHICKEN OREGON

Some of the best and tastiest mushrooms in the world are grown right here in America, in Oregon, and this dish takes full advantage of these wonderful, earthy vegetables. This quick and easy dish is fun to create—and eat. Just ask my family! It's a perfect meal after a hard day's work.

What you'll need:
- 3 tablespoons extra-virgin olive oil
- 16 medium white mushroom caps, rinsed
- 24 ounces skinless, boneless chicken breasts
  Juice of $1\frac{1}{2}$ lemons
- 1 sprig rosemary, cut
- 1 cup low-sodium chicken broth
  Salt and pepper to taste

What you'll do:
Heat a large skillet until drops of water sizzle in it. Add the oil, mushroom caps, and chicken and sauté the chicken and mushrooms until chicken is light brown on both sides. Add the lemon juice, rosemary, and chicken broth. Add salt and pepper to taste. Bring to a boil and serve.

Serves 4 (male-sized portions). Women: Slice off about 2 ounces chicken and set aside. Wrap in foil and eat for breakfast or add to lunch or dinner the next day.

"Just put on a pair of walking shoes, grab your keys, and go! A walk was never so easy before!"

—*The Daily Adele Dose*

• •

Date:

What I ate...for breakfast: _____

_____

_____

What I ate...for my morning hard-chew snacks: _____

_____

What I ate...for lunch: _____

_____

_____

_____

What I ate...for my afternoon soft chews: _____

What I ate...for dinner: _____

_____

_____

_____

How I felt: _____

_____

_____

How I kept moving: _____

_____

_____

What I drank: _____

_____

Did I use the tape measure correctly to calculate my lost inches?

_____

The Look Is in the Beholder

According to a June 1996 Newsweek *poll, the average woman is approximately 5'4" tall and weighs about 145 pounds. The average supermodel, on the other hand, is approximately 5'9" tall and weighs 110 pounds.*

Maybe it's time we stopped looking at the runway's impossible ideal as our goal. It's only setting oneself up for sabotage to try for a weight that's difficult to achieve—let alone maintain. Be more realistic in your weight-loss goals and you'll not only be healthier, mentally and physically, but you'll also have a lot more fun!

Don't feel like measuring? Simply pick out that one pair of pants or jeans you haven't been able to wear in years. Every month, notice how much looser they feel!

"The sky's the limit when it comes to 'Foods You Adore'—as long as you stick to my four rules outlined in The 5-Day Miracle Diet. You can have whatever 'Extras' you decide to eat!"

—*The Daily Adele Dose*

• •

Date:

What I ate...for breakfast: _____
_____
_____

What I ate...for my morning hard-chew snacks: _____
_____

What I ate...for lunch: _____
_____
_____
_____

What I ate...for my afternoon soft chews: _____

What I ate...for dinner: _____
_____
_____
_____

How I felt: _____
_____
_____

How I kept moving: _____
_____
_____

What I drank: _____
_____

Did I write down any "guilt feelings" I was having in my journal— and analyze them? _____

LIQUOR "LIE-SENSE"

Ask Melissa and she'll tell you that she's really shy. It's hard to believe that this human resources director at a major company, this confident, responsible, and attractive young woman, is shy.

But when she first came to see me, she was more than shy. She was tired. And about twenty pounds overweight. Over the next few months, Melissa no longer cared about her weight—although she lost the twenty pounds. She had more energy than she ever had before in her life!

But still there was that shyness, which contradicted her familial role as the clown, the funny, wild, crazy gal. The role followed her all the way through college and was still there now, in her new position as head of personnel.

To keep up "appearances," and hide her shyness, Melissa drank. A glass or two (or three) of Chardonnay and she became witty, clever, zany, the most charismatic person at the party.

The healthier Melissa became, however, the more she hated the idea of being "hooked" on alcohol to be herself. It was a *fathead* issue she wanted to destroy.

She decided to test the waters at her college reunion a few months back. Instead of wine or vodka, she drank sparkling water and *pretended* to be drunk. She merely relaxed and let the party flow around her.

Soon Melissa was having a great time. She was laughing. She was charming. She looked the sophisticated career woman she was— without a drop of blood-sugar-mayhem-making alcohol in her.

The result? She didn't overindulge at dinner. She enjoyed herself immensely. And she was there, in the moment, without a crutch.

The next week she came into my office smiling. Now, that's empowerment.

"Our ancestors didn't have late meetings, crucial deadlines, or rush-hour traffic. It's no wonder all this wear and tear on us means we need more vitamins and minerals to cope. The 5-Day Miracle Diet provides for this!"

—*The Daily Adele Dose*

• •

Date:

What I ate...for breakfast: _____
_____
_____

What I ate...for my morning hard-chew snacks: _____
_____

What I ate...for lunch: _____
_____
_____
_____

What I ate...for my afternoon soft chews: _____

What I ate...for dinner:_____
_____
_____
_____

How I felt: _____
_____
_____

How I kept moving: _____
_____
_____

What I drank: _____
_____

Is my current vitamin-mineral supplement providing all the nutrients I need? _____

LOOKIN' GOOD

The best way to exercise in the gym is au naturel, at least where your face is concerned. But if makeup is all that's stopping you from going to the gym during lunch, here are some ways to ensure you won't go back to the office looking like a mess:

- If you wear makeup at the gym, make sure it's oil-free. You don't want to clog any pores while you're working up a sweat.
- Choose smudgeproof or waterproof mascara.
- Keep eye shadow neutral in the office and at the gym.
- Spritz your face with water while exercising and when you're finished.
- If you're not going to shower right away, make sure you cleanse your skin with a cool-feeling toner. Use moist towelettes on your body to feel fresh.
- Remember to go simple all day long. Makeup that's appropriate in the office might look dirty under the gym's lights. Plus there's more chance for it to smudge, run, or fade.
- If you're not going to shampoo, spritz your hair with some water, then a bit of mousse. It will give you back some style—and you'll smell good, too!
- If you're a woman who is blessed with skin that doesn't need makeup—or a man (who just doesn't wear it)—you're one of the fortunate ones: Just take a quick shower, towel-dry your hair, glance in the mirror, and off you go!

"I might have been born in a box of cookies, but today I live in a world where there is nothing, not even chocolate, that will ever box me in again!"

—*The Daily Adele Dose*

• •

Date:

What I ate...for breakfast: _____

_____

_____

What I ate...for my morning hard-chew snacks: _____

_____

What I ate...for lunch: _____

_____

_____

_____

What I ate...for my afternoon soft chews: _____

What I ate...for dinner: _____

_____

_____

_____

How I felt: _____

_____

_____

How I kept moving: _____

_____

_____

What I drank: _____

_____

Did I wake up a little more energetic, a little less worried today?

_____

BREAK-FAST CREATIVELY

During the week, that slice of bread and low-fat cheese is enough as you run through the door. There's too much going on, too many errands, chores, deadlines.... Who has time to linger over breakfast and the paper?

Weekends are different. We all take a step back and (except when there are soccer games, grocery shopping, or plumbing emergencies) we get to relax a bit more.

Sometimes, we even sleep a bit later.

As you all know, the 5-Day Miracle Diet takes our different rhythms into account. From Early Bird to Midnight Owl, I've devised programs that keep your meals and hard chews timed exactly right.

Eating breakfast a little bit later is one thing, but eating the same thing? Yes, it can be boring—and that's the last thing the 5-Day Miracle Diet is all about. Here are some ways to put the punch back in breakfast, the fun back in lingering over herbal tea while you read the Sunday papers:

✔ Use a fresh piece of whole-grain bread. Spread it with your allotment of natural peanut butter. Actually place the bread on a dish, slice it in half, and serve with some herbal tea and lemon.

✔ Try my Winter White Omelet. It's a fabulous recipe that's made with egg whites and you'll find it within these pages.

✔ Place the thinnest slices of smoked salmon (as an occasional and different treat) on your slice of bread. Add lemon and capers for a delicious taste sensation.

✔ Eat your cereal (on alternate days) with a teaspoon. It will make it last longer and you'll savor every bite!

✔ Take a tip from Seinfeld's kitchen cupboard. Add variety to those cereal mornings. Try new brands. Switch to hot cereal, then back to cold. Mix them up for your own delicious brand. Hey, you never know. Mr. Kellogg just might come knocking on your door.

✔ Make breakfast an occasion. Concentrate on the environment instead of the food. Put on some soft jazz or a classical piece. Add some flowers on the table. Use a pretty dish to serve your food. Linger over herbal tea, decaf coffee, or ice-cold water.

"Choosing a healthy lifestyle is not a death sentence. It's a positive affirmation of yourself, of what you believe, and what you hold dear for your future!"

—*The Daily Adele Dose*

• •

Date:

What I ate...for breakfast: _____

_____

_____

What I ate...for my morning hard-chew snacks: _____

_____

What I ate...for lunch: _____

_____

_____

_____

What I ate...for my afternoon soft chews: _____

What I ate...for dinner: _____

_____

_____

_____

How I felt: _____

_____

_____

How I kept moving: _____

_____

_____

What I drank: _____

_____

Did I try an omelet made with three egg whites instead of the usual breakfast ?_____

WEEKLY ASSESSMENT

WEIGHTY ISSUES

Last week's weight: _____

Pounds lost: _____

New weight: _____

*Don't forget those lost ounces and half
pounds. They add up!*

. . . .

**Life might be a bowl of cherries for some people, but I'll
guarantee they aren't in good blood sugar.
A better cliché: Life is a bowl of apples—or carrots or
hot and straight-from-the-grill veggies!**

. . . .

A WEEK's "POCKETFUL OF MIRACLES"

This week, concentrate on the *natural* exercise you might have
done this week—without giving it another thought. Maybe you got off
your bus two stops sooner so that you could walk part of the way to
work. Maybe you took the stairs instead of the elevator from floor to
floor. Perhaps you took the dog on an extra long walk, circling the
whole park instead of just opening the door to the backyard. Or
maybe you simply laced up your walking shoes and decided to go out
for a brisk walk—just because it was a nice day. For someone whose
exercise in the past didn't go further than reaching for the chips, these
things are miracles indeed!

Here's a miracle from a client and a former couch potato:
•*When I came home from work on Tuesday, I actually* wanted *to go out
for a jog!*

Now it's your turn: _____

_____

_____

"Saboteurs are always ready to pounce. Be ready for them—by identifying and recognizing your fathead issues and breaking the link with a new form of action or thought!"

—The Daily Adele Dose

• •

Date:

What I ate...for breakfast: _____

_____

_____

What I ate...for my morning hard-chew snacks: _____

_____

What I ate...for lunch: _____

_____

_____

_____

What I ate...for my afternoon soft chews:_____

What I ate...for dinner:_____

_____

_____

_____

How I felt: _____

_____

_____

How I kept moving: _____

_____

_____

What I drank: _____

_____

*Did you give someone you love a hug today—instead of sharing a piece of cake?*_____

VEGETABLE LEGUME GRILL

This beautiful and delectable dish not only enhances grilled vegetables but also makes an entire meal of them. You can serve this dish hot or cold—which makes it perfect to eat the next day for lunch or dinner.

What you'll need:
- 4 cups canned fava beans, drained
- ¼ cup balsamic vinegar
- ¼ cup peeled and chopped white or red onions
- 2 tablespoons chopped thyme
- 1 tablespoon chopped basil
- 2 tablespoons extra-virgin olive oil
- Salt and pepper to taste
- Special Grilled Vegetables (page 140)

What you'll do:

Mix all the ingredients except the grilled vegetables in a container and cover with plastic wrap. Marinate for 1 hour.

Arrange the grilled vegetables on a flat dish. Spread the bean mixture over them. Serve hot or cold.

Serves 4 (male-sized) portions. Women: Spoon about ¼ cup beans into a container. Eat the next day at lunch or dinner with leftover grilled vegetables and a salad. Don't forget to add the oil toward your daily fat allotment.

> *"'Owning' the 5-Day Miracle Diet means that this is the way you eat most of the time—and less and less time passes when you are not eating this way!"*
>
> —*The Daily Adele Dose*

• •

Date:

What I ate...for breakfast: _____
_____
_____

What I ate...for my morning hard-chew snacks: _____
_____

What I ate...for lunch: _____
_____
_____
_____

What I ate...for my afternoon soft chews: _____

What I ate...for dinner: _____
_____
_____
_____

How I felt: _____
_____
_____

How I kept moving: _____
_____
_____

What I drank: _____
_____

Did I identify, recognize, and attack a fathead *today?* _____

WHAT A PEAR!

Pears make the perfect hard chew, but
many people don't opt for them for one
simple reason: They never seem ripe in the
store. One woman told me that she got confused
every time she walked past the produce. "There are just
too many varieties, and I'm not going to waste my hard chew on
something that won't taste good!"

She had a point. So I've included this small section on choosing
the right pear for your hard chew:

✔ Purchase pears while firm but not hard. Soften them up slightly in
a bowl at home. Too soft and the pear won't do its job!
✔ Pull at the stem. If it loosens easily, the pear is ripe.
✔ Scrub the pear gently to clean; don't rub the skin off.

The three most common pears and what they taste like:

• *Anjou* pears look almost like bell-shaped potatoes. They are very
sweet, with a firm texture.

• *Bartlett* pears are the yellow-green pears you see most often in
your grocery store. The more yellow they are, the riper they will be,
so stick with ones that have a green tone for a perfect hard chew.

• *Bosc* pears are similar in looks to the Anjou, but they are smaller.
Their taste is more tart than that of other pears.

"My life is an open book: I love to eat—and I've worked hard to devise a program where I can eat and feel absolutely fabulous at the same time!"

—*The Daily Adele Dose*

• •

Date:

What I ate...for breakfast: _____
_____

What I ate...for my morning hard-chew snacks: _____
_____

What I ate...for lunch: _____
_____
_____
_____

What I ate...for my afternoon soft chews: _____

What I ate...for dinner: _____
_____
_____
_____

How I felt: _____
_____
_____

How I kept moving: _____
_____
_____

What I drank: _____
_____

Did I stop a negative thought in its tracks by using logic and my new-found sense of stability? _____

"Before I discovered the 5-Day Miracle Diet, I was floundering. I started diets and quit within the first week. I dreamed of fitting into a smashing bathing suit, then never did anything about it. I berated myself, calling myself lazy and no good. What a difference! I've been on the program for three weeks and I haven't even wanted to call it quits. I feel great, ready to wear a bathing suit no matter what shape I'm in!"

—A fiftysomething bank manager and single mother of two

SLEEVELESS DRESSES: AT ANY AGE!

Yes, there is life after menopause. In fact, you can still do something about fat—a lot of something! One study found that postmenopausal women who had a sedentary lifestyle weighed twenty-seven pounds more than their premenopausal counterparts. But those postmenopausal women who exercised weighed only twelve more pounds than those younger and fitter!

"Making love to a person you love is much more satisfying than making love to a huge steak and fries!"

—*The Daily Adele Dose*

• •

Date: _____

What I ate...for breakfast: _____
_____
_____

What I ate...for my morning hard-chew snacks: _____
_____

What I ate...for lunch: _____
_____
_____
_____

What I ate...for my afternoon soft chews: _____

What I ate...for dinner: _____
_____
_____
_____

How I felt: _____
_____
_____

How I kept moving: _____
_____
_____

What I drank: _____
_____

Did I try one of the new side dish recipes in this book? _____

THE 5-DAY MIRACLE DIET GOES TO THE MOVIES

Perhaps it's the memories of Saturday afternoons in the cool air of the movies, gobbling popcorn and candy while you stared wide-eyed at the screen. Perhaps it's simply the smell of popping corn that brings your **Nostalgia *fathead*** to mind as you approach the theater. Or perhaps it's the advertisements strategically placed throughout the theater: From the walls to the screens, everything seems to shout "Movies and food go together like stars and directors."

Then again, it might be the fact that you've skipped dinner to go to an earlier movie, planning to have a repast after the show is over. Wrong! It's better to eat early than wait until 9:30 or 10:00. If you're with friends who love to dine in the moonlight hours, you can still join the fun without sacrificing your 5-Day Miracle Diet plan. Eat 1 ounce of protein and a hard chew in the movies. (Who will hear you anyway? Everyone's busy eating popcorn!) Later, at the restaurant, you can eat your remaining protein and your veggies. (It's my "two-thumbs-up" recommendation!)

Even if the **Nostalgic Habit *fathead*** refuses to go away, you can still enjoy the latest blockbuster without straying from the 5-Day Miracle Diet. Today, many theaters offer healthier, hot-air versions of their artery-clogging buttered popcorn. You can also get iced tea or bottled water instead of soda.

And, of course, there's always "BYOB": Bring your own (string) beans and crunch in peace.

"You can go on vacation, plan a holiday meal, or even enjoy those weeks between Thanksgiving and Christmas without getting into that 'Recess State of Mind.' Isn't it better to really experience all this excitement with your senses intact, your moods calm, and your energy in top form?"

—*The Daily Adele Dose*

• •

Date:

What I ate...for breakfast: _____

_____

_____

What I ate...for my morning hard-chew snacks: _____

_____

What I ate...for lunch: _____

_____

_____

_____

What I ate...for my afternoon soft chews: _____

What I ate...for dinner: _____

_____

_____

_____

How I felt: _____

_____

_____

How I kept moving: _____

_____

What I drank: _____

_____

Did I plan ahead for the holiday meal? _____

WHEN A CRAVING JUST WON'T QUIT

Red alert. Emergency situation. SOS. Maybe it's only the second day of your diet. Maybe it's a *fathead* issue calling out. Who cares. It doesn't matter. You want your candy/cookie/carbo/cheese now!

Wait!

Take a deep breath. Go to the "Quick Fix" list in *The 5-Day Miracle Diet* to help get you past your raging craving. Here's a list to help you out when a phone call to a friend, a walk around the block, or any other distraction just isn't going to work. Like the others, they'll give you a touch of that starchy sweetness you crave—without adding extra pounds or hurting your good blood sugar work.

- 1 slice honeydew
- ½ of a tangerine
- 2 unsalted pretzel rings
- 1 unsalted, unsweetened rice cake
- ½ slice whole-grain pita
- A handful of string beans
- A Chinese pear or any other hard chew
- Mint, lemon, or Sleepy Time herbal tea

"Motivation is only one small factor on the 5-Day Miracle Diet. By eating the right foods at the right time, you won't need motivation! Your good blood sugar will take care of it all!"

—*The Daily Adele Dose*

• •

Date:

What I ate...for breakfast: _____

_____

_____

What I ate...for my morning hard-chew snacks: _____

_____

What I ate...for lunch: _____

_____

_____

_____

What I ate...for my afternoon soft chews: _____

What I ate...for dinner: _____

_____

_____

_____

How I felt: _____

_____

_____

How I kept moving: _____

_____

_____

What I drank: _____

_____

Did I sip an unsweetened herb tea after dinner—and nothing else?

_____

TO EAT OR NOT TO EAT
AT YOUR BEST FRIEND'S WEDDING

If you are anything like me, celebrations are times of rejoicing—and times of rejoicing mean food. Weddings, in particular, are tempting, both to body chemistry and the **Emotional *fathead***, especially if the bride or groom in question is your best friend!

Here are a few things I've learned along the way to handle weddings, whether a sit-down banquet, a lavish buffet, or an artfully designed cocktail party.

- Eat a hard-chew snack before you step in the door. That apple, pear, or baby carrot will go far in keeping your body chemistry in check and your blood sugar balanced.

- Scope out the buffet before you dig in. Decide what looks really good and what you really want. Forget the rest. Believe me, no one's looking (unless it's your brother's wedding and your mother wishes you were getting married, too!).

- As soon as the waiter places the fruit cup in front of you, ask him or her to give you your salad with dressing on the side. This way, they'll have time to do as you ask before drenching 250 plates of greens.

- Use the wedding as a "Foods You Adore" occasion. Try to stay in good blood sugar at least two days before the event. Decide which is most important to you: the champagne, the poached salmon in rich, creamy dill sauce, or the mocha multilayered wedding cake. Can't decide? Have a bite of two—or all three! You can get back in good blood sugar tomorrow, especially if you plan a good long walk.

- This is the most important tip: Have fun! It's not every day that a wedding takes place. I promise you that if you're in good blood sugar, you won't be as tempted as you think. Even your *fathead* will be quieter. It simply doesn't have the chemical "fuel" to play games. Remember, this diet is for life, not a passing fad.

"I would no sooner go into an important business meeting in low blood sugar than I would go in dressed in jeans, with my hair dirty, or completely ill prepared!"

—*The Daily Adele Dose*

● ●

Date:

What I ate...for breakfast: _____

_____

_____

What I ate...for my morning hard-chew snacks: _____

_____

What I ate...for lunch: _____

_____

_____

_____

What I ate...for my afternoon soft chews: _____

What I ate...for dinner: _____

_____

_____

_____

How I felt: _____

_____

_____

How I kept moving: _____

_____

_____

What I drank: _____

_____

Did I get a new haircut as proof of the new me? _____

WEIGHTY ISSUES

Last week's weight: _____

Pounds lost: _____

New weight: _____

Don't forget those lost ounces and half pounds. They add up!

• •

Dance, jump, and raise your arms in triumph. No, these aren't impressions of the Olympics—they are you! The brand new, active person who takes pride in ordinary, everyday, 5-Day Miracle Diet, life.

• •

A WEEK'S "POCKETFUL OF MIRACLES"

Another week, another opportunity for miracles. By now you must be experiencing some of the fabulous benefits of the 5-Day Miracle Diet. It wouldn't surprise me if you suddenly had more energy, more focus, more of an even keel. Nor would it surprise me if you were also finding success in other areas of your life, in addition to your weight loss. Perhaps you're due for a promotion. Maybe you've met someone new. Or maybe it's simply the fact that you were spontaneous for the first time in your life, deciding to call a friend and go out to the movies at the last minute!

Whatever your miracle is, it's important to write it down and remember it in the week to come. Remembering some of the special things my diet has brought to your life will help you "own" it. Plus you'll have the added bonus of smiling whenever you think of your "miracle"!

Here's a miracle from a new client who'd recently read the book:
• *For the first time in my life, I didn't start my day with orange juice. By Day Five, I felt energized and I didn't miss it at all!*

Now it's your turn: _____

_____

_____

"How proud you feel! How strong, how vital, how confident!"

—*The Daily Adele Dose*

• •

Date:

What I ate...for breakfast: _____
_____
_____

What I ate...for my morning hard-chew snacks: _____
_____

What I ate...for lunch: _____
_____
_____
_____

What I ate...for my afternoon soft chews: _____

What I ate...for dinner: _____
_____
_____
_____

How I felt: _____
_____
_____

How I kept moving: _____
_____
_____

What I drank: _____
_____

Did I eat an optional roll at lunch today? _____

Artichokes Sienna

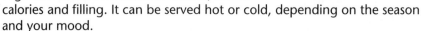

Someone once said that eating an artichoke is like getting to know a person really well. And this dish is certainly one that you will become well acquainted with. It's a perfect vegetable choice for lunch or dinner, low in calories and filling. It can be served hot or cold, depending on the season and your mood.

This particular artichoke recipe is rich in seasonings and can be eaten alone. Add a slice of low-fat cheese and a whole-grain roll and you will think you are in the Italian countryside, elegantly dining on sophisticated fare.

What you'll need:
- 4 medium-to-large artichokes
- 8–10 drops of fresh lemon juice
- 12 cloves garlic, crushed
- 2 teaspoons extra-virgin olive oil plus extra to sprinkle on cooked artichokes
- 3 sprigs of fresh Italian (flat-leaf) parsley, rinsed
- 8 coarsely chopped basil leaves
- Salt and pepper to taste

What you'll do:

Soak the artichokes in cold water for 30 minutes to clean. Shake off the excess water and snip off the spiky ends. Place the artichokes, stem side down, in a medium saucepan. Add the lemon juice, garlic, oil, parsley, and basil. Fill the saucepan with water until the artichokes are halfway covered. Add salt and pepper to taste and bring to a boil. Cover the saucepan and simmer for 30 minutes, or until you can easily pull off an artichoke leaf.

Place an artichoke in each of four bowls. Open each artichoke like a flower. Sprinkle the artichokes with olive oil and water. Serve.

If you prefer, cover the artichokes and place them in the refrigerator for several hours to serve cold.

Serves 4 as a lunch or dinner veggie—not as a hard chew!

"The psychological, emotional reasons you reach for food can be unique, as you are. The key is to recognize them and change them in ways that are right for you!"

—*The Daily Adele Dose*

• •

Date:

What I ate...for breakfast: _____
_____
_____

What I ate...for my morning hard-chew snacks: _____
_____

What I ate...for lunch: _____
_____
_____
_____

What I ate...for my afternoon soft chews: _____

What I ate...for dinner: _____
_____
_____
_____

How I felt: _____
_____
_____

How I kept moving: _____
_____
_____

What I drank: _____
_____

Did I tell the waiter to take away the rolls before I was tempted to eat one? _____

THE OFFICE IS (ABSOLUTELY) A PLACE FOR CARROTS!

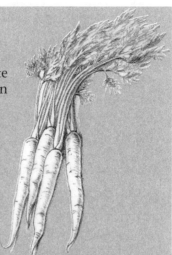

Okay. Perhaps it isn't entirely appropriate to munch on your carrots if you're sitting in your three-piece suit conducting a meeting that could end up in a six-figure deal. But there are ways to sneak in your hard-chew snacks within your two-hour time limit without anyone even knowing. Here are some tips:

✔ Excuse yourself from the meeting for a moment. Instead of going to the restroom, go to your office and eat your hard-chew snacks!
✔ Make eating your hard-chew snacks the very first thing you do when you reach the office. This way you've taken care of business *before* business starts.

"I feel empowered. It's as simple as that: empowerment. That's what the 5-Day Miracle Diet gives you—in spades!"

—*The Daily Adele Dose*

• •

Date: _____

What I ate...for breakfast: _____
_____
_____

What I ate...for my morning hard-chew snacks: _____
_____

What I ate...for lunch: _____
_____
_____
_____

What I ate...for my afternoon soft chews: _____

What I ate...for dinner: _____
_____
_____
_____

How I felt: _____
_____
_____

How I kept moving: _____
_____
_____

What I drank: _____
_____

Did I try grilling my veggies or my protein today? _____

THE TOP TEN "MIRACLES" YOU'LL FIND IN THE 5-DAY MIRACLE DIET

1. More energy

2. A calm, centered manner

3. Confidence

4. Empowerment: standing up for yourself

5. A zest for life

6. Better concentration

7. Disappearance of food cravings

8. Weight loss

9. A sparkle in your eyes and a glow to your cheeks

10. A sense of well-being you've never had before!

"Don't let people say you have an eating disorder. It's chemical, pure and simple, and five days will balance your blood sugar and stop the 'crave faze' problem once and for all!"

—*The Daily Adele Dose*

• •

Date:

What I ate...for breakfast: _____

_____

_____

What I ate...for my morning hard-chew snacks: _____

_____

What I ate...for lunch: _____

_____

_____

_____

What I ate...for my afternoon soft chews: _____

What I ate...for dinner: _____

_____

_____

_____

How I felt: _____

_____

_____

How I kept moving: _____

_____

_____

What I drank: _____

_____

Did I eat a soft or hard chew before walking into the restaurant—just in case I didn't get served right away? _____

LATE FOR WORK?

You might not be able to pet the cat, but you can stay with the 5-Day Miracle Diet.

Simply grab a quick, appropriate breakfast as you run out the door. Who cares if you run down the block chewing a slice of bread and a piece of low-fat cheese? Or a slice of chicken with a slice of bread? Easy, portable, and absolutely unobtrusive!

VEGETABLES CAN BE FUN!

Okay, so they're not a trip to Paris or a ride in the country. But vegetables don't have to be hours of drudgery, either!

Cut up your vegetables up to three days in advance. Put your hard-chew amounts in those new small perforated vegetable bags. They'll keep fresh until you're ready to chew. You'll lose some nutrients, but if you don't cut them up, you won't eat them at all! Remember, convenience is the key to keep you on track.

"Go slow. All the wonderful, positive 'miracles' will happen to your mind, body, and soul. But give yourself time. Attitudes took a long time to become ingrained—and it takes time to 'un-grain' them!"

—*The Daily Adele Dose*

• •

Date:

What I ate...for breakfast: _____
_____
_____

What I ate...for my morning hard-chew snacks: _____
_____

What I ate...for lunch: _____
_____
_____
_____

What I ate...for my afternoon soft chews: _____

What I ate...for dinner: _____
_____
_____
_____

How I felt: _____
_____
_____

How I kept moving: _____
_____
_____

What I drank: _____
_____

*Did I get enough sleep last night, so I won't hear the **Overtired fathead**?* _____

STRIPED BASS AND SUN-DRIED TOMATO EUROPA

The bright colors, scrumptious textures, and delectable taste of this dish make me happy to prepare it and serve it to my friends and family. And the nutritionist in me is even happier because the dish also combines unusual ingredients that are extremely high in essential fatty acids, vitamins, and minerals—without sacrificing great taste! It is slightly tart, which makes it a perfect foil for couscous. Serve with steamed slivers of zucchini, summer squash, and carrots.

What you'll need:
1/4 cup extra-virgin olive oil
24 ounces striped bass fillet
 8 cloves garlic, sliced
 3 ounces sun-dried tomatoes, cut in julienne strips
   Salt and pepper to taste
 1 bunch arugula, rinsed and coarsely chopped

What you'll do:
   Heat a large skillet until drops of water sizzle in its center. Add the oil and the fillet, skin side up, and sauté fillet until golden brown, about 2 minutes. Turn the fillet, add the garlic, and sauté until the garlic is golden brown. Add the sun-dried tomatoes, 1/2 cup water, salt, and pepper to taste and bring to a boil. Reduce the heat to low and simmer for 7 minutes. Add the arugula and bring to a boil for 3 minutes. Serve.

Serves four (male-sized portions). Women: Slice off about 2 ounces fish and put aside. Wrap in foil and eat for breakfast or add to lunch or dinner the next day.

"You might have been born sucking on a lollipop, but today you could care less about sugar. You're living in a fabulous world of health and well-being!"

—*The Daily Adele Dose*

• •

Date:

What I ate...for breakfast: _____
_____
_____

What I ate...for my morning hard-chew snacks: _____
_____

What I ate...for lunch: _____
_____
_____
_____

What I ate...for my afternoon soft chews: _____

What I ate...for dinner: _____
_____
_____
_____

How I felt: _____
_____
_____

How I kept moving: _____
_____
_____

What I drank: _____
_____

Did I decide how I'm going to handle an upcoming party? _____

Losing one pound a week translates into fifty-two pounds a year.

Just think: If you had started the 5-day Miracle Diet last year, you would already be about fifty pounds thinner!

AN OPEN LETTER

Dear Adele,

    I would like to thank you ahead of time for saving my life. I truly believe this is the answer that I have been searching for. As I have read your book, I am astonished by your thoughts on how to lose weight. I have done everything possible to find the answer. I am so confident that the 5-Day Miracle Diet will work for me, even though this is my first day. I know it is written for me.

—A thirtysomething woman who has only just begun

"Imagine: No more slave to cookies. No more fugitive from pasta prison. With my diet plan, you can hold your head up high and say, 'I can eat anything I want—because I, not my blood sugar, am in control of who I am and what I do!'"

—*The Daily Adele Dose*

• •

Date:

What I ate...for breakfast: _____

_____

_____

What I ate...for my morning hard-chew snacks: _____

_____

What I ate...for lunch: _____

_____

_____

_____

What I ate...for my afternoon soft chews: _____

What I ate...for dinner: _____

_____

_____

_____

How I felt: _____

_____

_____

How I kept moving: _____

_____

_____

What I drank: _____

_____

Did I make sure I got at least one hard chew in before dinner?

_____

Six months have almost come and gone, and with them a profound sense of achievement. In only six months, you, too, have changed—you, too, have seen knowledge and self-esteem "come" and weight issues "go."

Congratulations are in order, although it all probably seems so effortless to you now that you don't even realize what a tremendous accomplishment it is! You might even be thinking, "Why didn't I do this *sooner*?"

It's most likely difficult to remember what you were like before you started my program. Who was that sluggish, sad person who didn't like himself or herself very much? Not you. Not anymore. Although this is the last month you'll be writing in this particular journal, keep it up. There's no reason why you can't go out and buy a notebook and start with Month Seven. There's always something to learn about yourself, something wonderful, something startling, but always something special—because it concerns you.

And always remember that despite my guidance, despite my hints and insights and help, you are the one who did it. You are the one who took hold of your life and changed it. You are the one who made the 5-Day Miracle Diet your own; you were ready to embrace the joys, the energies, the new zest for life that had always been inside, lying dormant, waiting for you to take a stand.

And so, let the miracles begin—again and again!

Inch-by-Inch

Bust/chest: _____   Upper arms: _____

Wrists: _____   Waist: _____

Abdomen: _____   Hips and buttocks: _____

IN A WORD...

Sum up your monthly experience in one or two words. Use it as your "mantra" in the month to come. It's easy now that you've made the 5-Day Miracle Diet yours to keep! Here's one of my favorites:

I own the diet, and no one can take it away from me!

What's your good word?

_____

Shout it out. You should feel proud!

Life is a rich, full banquet. A loving relationship, a special place, a warm fire on a cold night, fireworks on the Fourth of July. Eating is only a part of all these experiences. Taste everything on the table and savor every bite!

You need specific ingredients to build a house that's strong and steady.

A diet is no different. Get low blood sugar under control, and your foundation is in place. Wow . . . what a beautiful house!

WEEKLY ASSESSMENT

WEIGHTY ISSUES

Last week's weight: _____

Pounds lost: _____

New weight: _____

Don't forget those lost ounces and half pounds. They add up!

• •

Here's a practical hint: When you make your plane reservation, tell them you want a special low-fat plate.
Most of the time these dishes are fresher, and you'll be served first while others are stuck with "airline food."

• •

A WEEK'S "POCKETFUL OF MIRACLES"

*T*his week, think about the actual concept called a "miracle."
No, I'm not talking about walking on water. I'm not talking about fishes and loaves. But I am talking about those daily, day-in-and-day-out ordinary experiences that can be quite extraordinary to the right person. For example, if you are trying to quit smoking, going a full day without a cigarette is quite an accomplishment, especially if you didn't think about puffing away the whole time. The same holds true for food. If you're a true "food sensualist" with some complex *fathead* issues, bypassing an overstuffed sandwich at a party is a miracle, especially if it didn't even *occur* to you to take a bite! Here's a miracle from a woman who'd written me after reading *The 5-Day Miracle Diet:*

• *On Day Four of the diet, I actually woke up without thinking about food. Would you believe it's the first time in my life?*

Now it's your turn: _____

_____

_____

"Eating seconds is second-rate. It's your blood sugar talking, not you."

—*The Daily Adele Dose*

• •

Date:

What I ate...for breakfast: _____
_____
_____

What I ate...for my morning hard-chew snacks: _____
_____

What I ate...for lunch: _____
_____
_____
_____

What I ate...for my afternoon soft chews: _____

What I ate...for dinner: _____
_____
_____
_____

How I felt: _____
_____
_____

How I kept moving: _____
_____
_____

What I drank: _____
_____

Did I remember to pack my hard-chew plastic bags in my attaché case today? _____

WALNUT SPINACH

This side dish is a marvelous and unusual accompaniment to my Endive Étoile (page 70). The small amount of walnuts adds a crunchy counterpart to the sweet spinach. It's a treat for your taste buds without sacrificing low-fat or low-caloric value. Add your allotment of protein, such as tuna or low-fat cheese, and you have a spectacular entrée that is suitable for either lunch or dinner.

What you'll need:
2 cups spinach leaves, stems removed
1 tablespoon extra-virgin olive oil
2 tablespoons chopped walnuts
½ teaspoon chopped garlic
½ cup low-fat chicken broth
   Salt and pepper to taste

What you'll do:
   Wash the spinach well. Cook in a 4-quart saucepan with only a teaspoon or two of water. The spinach will become soft and watery as it cooks.
   Drain the spinach and chop into medium-sized chunks. Set aside.
   Heat the oil in a skillet. Add the walnuts and garlic and sauté for 2 minutes over medium heat. Add the spinach and sauté another 2 minutes. Add the chicken broth and simmer for 3 minutes.
   Add salt and pepper to taste. Serve.

Serves 4. Don't forget to add the fat to your daily allotment.

"Remember, food is only as powerful as you make it!"

—The Daily Adele Dose

• •

Date:

What I ate...for breakfast: _____

_____

_____

What I ate...for my morning hard-chew snacks: _____

_____

What I ate...for lunch: _____

_____

_____

_____

What I ate...for my afternoon soft chews: _____

What I ate...for dinner: _____

_____

_____

_____

How I felt: _____

_____

_____

How I kept moving: _____

_____

_____

What I drank: _____

_____

Did I take a break from stress with a quick relaxation exercise?

_____

MIRROR, MIRROR ON THE WALL

Sometimes our motivation needs a jolt to get recharged. The best jolts come from those "ever-ready" photographs we have stuck in albums, in files, and in the kitchen drawer.

And the best way to keep those memories fresh is to take a picture of yourself every month. Yes, every month, in the same room, in the same chair or against the same wall.

You'll immediately see the difference in the way you look now and then. Perhaps there's more confidence in your smile, a gleam in your eye. Maybe you're wearing a nicer outfit now. You like being well groomed because you like yourself!

Seeing who you were—and who you are now—is the best motivation you can find for sticking to the 5-Day Miracle Diet this month and every month!

CAN'T YOU TAKE A RIBBING?

The look of the day in Victorian times was the hourglass shape. But it was far from natural: It is anatomically impossible to achieve this look without some kind of enhancement. This meant the searing pain of a tightly tied corset, which sometimes cut off so much of a woman's circulation that it resulted in stomach and respiratory trouble. Another solution was to simply remove a rib. It instantly made a woman's waist "waspish."

"Here's to your lifelong romance with good health, vitality, strength, confidence—and the 5-Day Miracle Diet!"

—*The Daily Adele Dose*

• •

Date:

What I ate...for breakfast: _____

_____

What I ate...for my morning hard-chew snacks: _____

_____

What I ate...for lunch: _____

_____

_____

_____

What I ate...for my afternoon soft chews: _____

What I ate...for dinner: _____

_____

_____

_____

How I felt: _____

_____

_____

How I kept moving: _____

_____

_____

What I drank: _____

_____

Did I reward myself today with a luxurious bath or a new computer toy? _____

SHALLOT CRÈME MUSHROOMS

Mushrooms make a wonderful palate for any number of herbs, spices, and cheeses. They are low in calories and enrich other ingredients with their own warm, earthy burst of flavor. These stuffed mushrooms are unusual. Egg whites take the place of heavy cream without sacrificing flavor. The result is a light, scrumptious appetizer or side dish to please a family or a crowd.

What you'll need:
- 24 cremini or large white mushroom caps, cleaned (save the stems)
  Salt and pepper to taste
- 1–2 tablespoons extra-virgin olive oil
- 1 cup chopped scallions
- ½ cup chopped onions
- ¼ cup chopped shallots
- 12 basil leaves, chopped
- 1 tablespoon chopped parsley
- 1 tablespoon grated low-fat Parmesan or Romano cheese
- 2 egg whites, lightly beaten

What you'll do:
Preheat the oven to 400° F.
Chop the mushroom stems. Set aside.
Place the mushrooms in a shallow baking dish and sprinkle with salt and pepper to taste. Bake in oven for 10 minutes.
Remove the mushrooms from the oven, drain, and set aside.

To make the stuffing:
Heat a 4-quart saucepan over high heat until drops of water sizzle in its center. Add the oil, scallions, onions, shallots, basil, parsley, and chopped mushroom stems.
Turn the heat down to low and sauté until all ingredients are soft, about 5 minutes. Remove the saucepan from the stove. Add salt and pepper to taste, the grated cheese, and the egg whites and stir.
Fill each mushroom with a tablespoon of stuffing. Return the baking dish to the oven and bake 6 minutes at 400° F. Serve.

Makes 4 servings of 6 mushrooms each. Don't forget to add the oil to your daily allotment of fat.

"Remember, it's not how close together you eat your meals that's important, but how far apart!"

—*The Daily Adele Dose*

• •

Date:

What I ate...for breakfast: _____
_____
_____

What I ate...for my morning hard-chew snacks: _____
_____

What I ate...for lunch: _____
_____
_____
_____

What I ate...for my afternoon soft chews: _____

What I ate...for dinner: _____
_____
_____
_____

How I felt: _____
_____
_____

How I kept moving: _____
_____
_____

What I drank: _____
_____

Did I eat my second hard-chew or soft-chew snack before my eight o'clock dinner? _____

AN APPLE A DAY

We know that apples make a great hard chew. They're portable, fresh, and easy to eat, and they even taste sweet.

But seriously, folks, there is life after Macs and Delicious. In fact, there's a whole world of apples out there, each one with its own unique crunch, flavor, and burst of taste!

Just to give your hard-chew palate some variety, here are some other apples you might want to try:

- *Granny Smith* are green, tart, and very crisp.

- *Jonathan Red* are small, bright red, and sweet.

- *Macoun.* The gourmet's delight. This variety is wine red, crisp, with a heavenly burst of flavor.

- *Northern Spy* are pale green and spicy, with a juicy tartness.

- *Rome Beauty* are large, dark red, and very sweet.

- *Golden Russet* are dusty red and sweet.

- *Gravenstein* are yellow, tart, and crisp.

- *Winesap* are small and spicy, with a burst of flavor.

"When you're in good blood sugar, all it takes is the first half a day each morning to stabilize your blood sugar. After each lunch, all you have to do is maintain it. That's it!"

—The Daily Adele Dose

Date:

What I ate...for breakfast: _____

What I ate...for my morning hard-chew snacks: _____

What I ate...for lunch: _____

What I ate...for my afternoon soft chews: _____

What I ate...for dinner: _____

How I felt: _____

How I kept moving: _____

What I drank: _____

Did I eat a few hors d'oeuvres and call it my entrée at a party?

_____

EXERCISE YOUR MIND

A paradox of life: When it comes to a deadline at work, we wouldn't miss it on penalty of death. Nor would we miss a dear friend's wedding or a big birthday bash for someone we love—even if we had a raging fever. But when it comes to ourselves? Forget about it.

Especially when it comes to exercise. "Oh, I just don't have time." "I couldn't fit it in." "I'm too tired." You know the rap.

But here's the Big Question: You wouldn't miss an important meeting at work, so why don't you treat exercise the same way?

Write your anticipated schedules down in your book, with the exact times and days you plan on burning those calories. Pretend it's one of those events you can't miss. And guess what? It is!

Time for "being good to yourself" is the most important appointment you'll ever have in life. It's a sobering thought, but true. If you don't take care of yourself, you can eventually forget all those parties, those deadlines, and those obligations.

Start now. This week. Write down your exercise time on the opposite page right now!

"This is the last diet you will ever need—or want!"
                                        —The Daily Adele Dose

• •

Date:

What I ate...for breakfast: _____
_____
_____

What I ate...for my morning hard-chew snacks: _____
_____

What I ate...for lunch: _____
_____
_____
_____

What I ate...for my afternoon soft chews: _____

What I ate...for dinner: _____
_____
_____
_____

How I felt: _____
_____
_____

How I kept moving: _____
_____
_____

What I drank: _____
_____

Did I make sure that I ate my hard chews at specific times, instead of nibbling on my carrots the whole day long? _____

A VEGGIE MIRACLE
WHIPPED UP IN FIVE MINUTES—OR LESS

Purchase pre-sliced vegetables. Add some tofu, roasted chicken (without the skin), turkey, or water-packed tuna and a drop of canola oil in a wok or large skillet, and voilà! A fabulous dinner in minutes for those nights when all you want to do is collapse.

• •

"Popcorn used to be my best friend. Now it's **The 5-Day Miracle Diet** *book!"*

—A woman whom I met and helped on **The Gordon Elliott Show**

• •

> *"Live your life. Love your life. Thanks to the 5-Day Miracle Diet, you have the power!"*
>
> —*The Daily Adele Dose*

• •

Date:

What I ate...for breakfast: _____

_____

_____

What I ate...for my morning hard-chew snacks: _____

_____

What I ate...for lunch: _____

_____

_____

_____

What I ate...for my afternoon soft chews: _____

What I ate...for dinner: _____

_____

_____

_____

How I felt: _____

_____

_____

How I kept moving: _____

_____

_____

What I drank: _____

_____

Did I find myself smiling today—for no good reason? _____

WEEKLY ASSESSMENT

WEIGHTY ISSUES

Last week's weight: ————————————

Pounds lost: ————————————

New weight: ————————————

Don't forget those lost ounces and half pounds. They add up!

• •

Think about it. You were born a miracle—and you can return to your "roots" with the 5-Day Miracle Diet's physiological basics.

• •

A WEEK'S "POCKETFUL OF MIRACLES"

*I*t's time to concentrate on food issues—and food miracles. You've been on the 5-Day Miracle Diet for some time now and you know the routine by heart. You've even begun to understand why your particular *fathead* exists—and you've been fighting a winning battle.

To help in your resolve, think of some food habit that has changed, something that has to be a miracle because you'd never been able to do it before now!

Here's an example from a pleased client who knows that the miracles are all inside him:

•*Last night, for the first time, I ordered my burger and, without thinking, pushed aside the fries and asked for a salad instead. I didn't even have any desire for the fries. I really wanted my salad. I wanted my greens!*

Now it's your turn: ————————————————

————————————————————————————————

————————————————————————————————

"Don't unconsciously space out when you eat. Write it all down. You just may forget the peanuts on the plane or the cookie you nibbled on the way out of the house— which can stop your good blood sugar from stabilizing!"

—*The Daily Adele Dose*

Date:

What I ate...for breakfast: _____
_____
_____

What I ate...for my morning hard-chew snacks: _____
_____

What I ate...for lunch: _____
_____
_____
_____

What I ate...for my afternoon soft chews: _____

What I ate...for dinner: _____
_____
_____
_____

How I felt: _____
_____
_____

How I kept moving: _____
_____
_____

What I drank: _____
_____

Have I looked at an old picture of myself today—amazed at the positive changes I've made? _____

Appetizing Appetizers

Those cute little mushroom caps, that elegant salmon with sour cream and capers, the mouthwatering baked Brie...these appetizers are not just designed to taunt you.

Nor are they a ploy to get you to eat even more than you planned—if you know what you're doing.

I've long been a fan of the most amazing, delicious appetizers, which become my main meal. Three or four of these delicacies and you have a complete meal, without over-sized restaurant portions that are notorious for too much protein, pasta, sugar, and fat.

Hors d'oeuvres can be an excellent way to go at weddings, bar and bat mitzvahs, and business conferences, too. Scout out the table. Put a delicate three or four items on your plate, and yes, you have a marvelous dinner! Yum.

"Maintaining the 5-Day Miracle Diet is easy. Sure, part of it is adding more food, but the bulk of it is living each day, loving each day, 'owning' each day!"

—*The Daily Adele Dose*

• •

Date:

What I ate...for breakfast: _____

_____

_____

What I ate...for my morning hard-chew snacks: _____

_____

What I ate...for lunch: _____

_____

_____

_____

What I ate...for my afternoon soft chews: _____

What I ate...for dinner: _____

_____

_____

_____

How I felt: _____

_____

_____

How I kept moving: _____

_____

_____

What I drank: _____

_____

Did I watch my protein allotment today? _____

SIZZLING SWORDFISH

Use only the freshest swordfish in this delectable dish, one that makes me rhapsodic about the sea. Spices and herbs make it a piquant dish, one worthy of a King or Queen Neptune. Serve with steamed rice, broccoli, and my Special Grilled Vegetables (page 140) for a plate that is as colorful as it is delicious.

What you'll need:
- 4 tablespoons extra-virgin olive oil
- 24 ounces swordfish fillets
- 2 large red bell peppers, sliced very thin
- 1 medium onion, sliced very thin
- 8 finely chopped basil leaves
- 2 cloves finely chopped garlic
- 1/4 teaspoon fresh chopped thyme or 1/8 teaspoon dried
- Salt and pepper to taste
- 1/2 cup balsamic vinegar
- 1/2 cup bottled water

What you'll do:
Heat a large skillet until drops of water sizzle in its center. Add 2 tablespoons of the olive oil and the swordfish and sauté the fish for 2 minutes on each side. Remove and set aside.

Using the same pan, add the remaining oil and the peppers, onions, basil, garlic, and thyme. Add salt and pepper to taste. Sauté ingredients over medium heat, stirring often, until vegetables are light brown.

Add the balsamic vinegar and water to the mixture and bring to a boil. Return the swordfish to the mixture and boil for 6 minutes over low heat. Serve.

Serves 4 (male-sized portions). Women: Slice off about 2 ounces fish and eat for lunch or dinner the next day. Don't forget to add the oil toward your fat intake for the day.

MIRACLE DIET CHEF'S HINT: Purchase a small pair of cooking scissors. Use them exclusively to snip and chop fresh herbs.

"Empowerment: It's the feeling you have when you stand up for what you want. And it starts with a simple 'No, please take this back. It's not what I ordered' in a restaurant!"

—*The Daily Adele Dose*

Date:

What I ate...for breakfast: _____
_____
_____

What I ate...for my morning hard-chew snacks: _____
_____

What I ate...for lunch: _____
_____
_____
_____

What I ate...for my afternoon soft chews: _____

What I ate...for dinner: _____
_____
_____
_____

How I felt: _____
_____
_____

How I kept moving: _____
_____
_____

What I drank: _____
_____

*Did I weigh my food once, and only once, so I could get an idea of my portion size?*_____

DID YOU KNOW...

Butter and margarine have exactly the same calories—and both have been found to have cholesterol-building properties in some people. So when you decide to have a "Food You Adore," go for the gold...butter, that is!

Walk Your Way to Fitness

There's always a good excuse waiting when it comes to not doing exercise. From "It's raining" and "I'm uncoordinated" to "I'm too out of shape" and "I don't know how," there's a rationale for not doing any kind of physical activity.

But there's one exercise that has no viable excuse: walking. Everyone can do it, in any shape or condition, and in any kind of weather (you can do it inside, on a treadmill, or at the mall). All you need is a good pair of shoes and a half hour of your time.

Some studies show you can even get the cardiovascular and fat-burning benefits if you break it up: walk only fifteen minutes in the morning and fifteen minutes at night.

So what's your excuse?

"For every day you stick with the 5-Day Miracle Diet, you will feel better and better!"

—*The Daily Adele Dose*

• •

Date:

What I ate...for breakfast: _____

_____

_____

What I ate...for my morning hard-chew snacks: _____

_____

What I ate...for lunch: _____

_____

_____

_____

What I ate...for my afternoon soft chews: _____

What I ate...for dinner: _____

_____

_____

_____

How I felt: _____

_____

_____

How I kept moving: _____

_____

_____

What I drank: _____

_____

Did I pack my lunch for the next day before I went to sleep?

_____

A Hard-Chew Reminder

Timing doesn't have to be a complicated process on the 5-Day Miracle Diet. Nor do you have to look at your watch every few minutes to make sure you haven't missed a hard-chew deadline. Keep a timer on your desk. Set it for two hours and voilà! You won't miss a beat.

WORTH A THOUSAND WORDS!

Find an old picture of what you used to look like: the worse, the better! Then take a photo now: See how great you look—happy and full of energy!

Who says you haven't made progress?

"You call this a diet? I call it a dream come true!"

—*The Daily Adele Dose*

• •

Date: _____

What I ate...for breakfast: _____
_____
_____

What I ate...for my morning hard-chew snacks: _____
_____

What I ate...for lunch: _____
_____
_____
_____

What I ate...for my afternoon soft chews: _____

What I ate...for dinner: _____
_____
_____
_____

How I felt: _____
_____
_____

How I kept moving: _____
_____
_____

What I drank: _____
_____

Did I try one of the new salad dressings found in this book?
_____

PARTY FAVORS

Although you might not quite believe it yet, parties can still be fabulous and fun while you're living on the 5-Day Miracle Diet. Here's how:

✔ Let everyone else go to the buffet table first. By the time you get there, it won't look as appetizing.
✔ Just say no when a waiter approaches with an hors d'oeuvre tray. He or she will be long gone before you even get a tempting whiff.
✔ Order a Virgin Mary extra hot. The spiciness will give you a buzz.
✔ Eat a hard chew before you walk in the door. It will make you feel full, balanced, and less tempted by the party food.
✔ If you hear the music, get up and dance!

- -

Jello Is Not the Only Fun Food

"The cherry tomato is a marvelous invention, producing as it does a satisfactorily explosive squish when bitten."

—**Miss Manners**

- -

"Watching your fat is healthy. Making it an obsession every time you put a morsel into your mouth is not! Remember what the Greeks believed: 'Moderation in all things.' And they were around for a long, long time!"

—*The Daily Adele Dose*

• •

Date: _____

What I ate...for breakfast: _____

_____

_____

What I ate...for my morning hard-chew snacks: _____

_____

What I ate...for lunch: _____

_____

_____

_____

What I ate...for my afternoon soft chews: _____

What I ate...for dinner: _____

_____

_____

_____

How I felt: _____

_____

_____

How I kept moving: _____

_____

_____

What I drank: _____

_____

Did I read my food labels when I went shopping? _____

A HARD-CHEW MÉLANGE

So you've had it with your baby carrots or apple, red cabbage or broccoli. Maybe you want to jazz things up just for variety's sake. Or maybe you happen to have a little bit of cabbage left, one carrot, and one broccoli floret and you don't want to waste them. No problem! Put them all in a little bag and eat a hard-chew salad. As long as you get those pituitary glands working and the blood chemistry balanced, it doesn't matter what kind of hard-chew vegetable you eat.

But remember: The hard chews *have* to be hard chews, like the crunchy, nutritious, fresh ones I list in my book, *The 5-Day Miracle Diet*. And they have to be eaten at the correct times.

That's all there is to it. Get those hard chews in at the right time and you are doing great! Whether they're solo or a mélange, you'll definitely be a hard-chew hero!

"When it comes to fat, use your judgment. A dollop brushed on your salad. A small amount on your entrée—which you can wipe off. An olive or a tiny piece of avocado in your vinegar-dressed salad. You didn't get fat by eating a little fat."

—*The Daily Adele Dose*

• •

Date:

What I ate...for breakfast: _____

_____

_____

What I ate...for my morning hard-chew snacks: _____

_____

What I ate...for lunch: _____

_____

_____

_____

What I ate...for my afternoon soft chews: _____

What I ate...for dinner: _____

_____

_____

_____

How I felt: _____

_____

_____

How I kept moving: _____

_____

_____

What I drank: _____

_____

Did I get a good night's sleep and wake up ready to face the new day—refreshed and raring to go? _____

WEEKLY ASSESSMENT

WEIGHTY ISSUES

Last week's weight: _____

Pounds lost: _____

New weight: _____

Don't forget those lost ounces and half pounds. They add up!

• •

The more weight you lose, the less your feet will ache after an exhausting day. And your back will thank you, too!

• •

A WEEK'S "POCKETFUL OF MIRACLES"

The pages are almost all filled in. Only a few more weeks to go. It's hard to believe that almost six months ago you began this journal feeling very different from the way you feel now. Way back then, you were probably a bit more tired, a bit more harried, and a little more moody. Sure, you were hopeful—but very, very cautious. After all, you've heard it before. Done it. Seen it. But you did have that extra ounce of anticipation. The 5-Day Miracle Diet was different. Maybe you really would lose weight and feel better than you ever had in your life. As you approach the end, these "miracles" are more important than ever. Don't lose your resolve or your good work. Remember when!

Here's a miracle to jog your memory; it's from a client:
• *For the first time in my life, I complained to a waiter. I told him that I had ordered my salad with dressing on the side—and that's what I wanted. Not greens literally wilted in a downpour of globby dressing!*

Now it's your turn: _____

_____

_____

"Food never solved any problem. Instead, concentrate on what's bothering you and face it directly."

—*The Daily Adele Dose*

• •

Date: _____

What I ate...for breakfast: _____
_____
_____

What I ate...for my morning hard-chew snacks: _____
_____

What I ate...for lunch: _____
_____
_____
_____

What I ate...for my afternoon soft chews: _____

What I ate...for dinner: _____
_____
_____
_____

How I felt: _____
_____
_____

How I kept moving: _____
_____
_____

What I drank: _____
_____

Did I try a new fish recipe today? _____

FIRE SCALE!

Here are some ways to keep the scale a tool—and keep you from being its slave:

1. Weigh yourself only once a week. At the same time. Wearing the same clothing.

2. Forget that old saw about "a good hard look at the mirror" with all your clothes off. *No one* looks good in stark light in a stark mirror. Maybe not even Demi Moore! Besides, unless you live in a nudist colony, the world doesn't see you like this. Instead, look at yourself in a smashing outfit. Before work. Before a party. See yourself looking groomed, confident, and chic. Proof that numbers only have power if you give in to them!

"When I'm in bad blood sugar, everything talks to me. The Chinese noodles. The pastries in the bakery. The chunky chicken salads at the deli. They whisper. They talk. They wave. They croon. But when I'm in good blood sugar, forget it. I don't even know they exist!"

—*The Daily Adele Dose*

Date:

What I ate...for breakfast: _____

_____

What I ate...for my morning hard-chew snacks: _____

_____

What I ate...for lunch: _____

_____

_____

_____

What I ate...for my afternoon soft chews: _____

What I ate...for dinner: _____

_____

_____

_____

How I felt: _____

_____

_____

How I kept moving: _____

_____

_____

What I drank: _____

_____

Did I try a different variety of rice? _____

HAVE IT YOUR WAY

The next time your kids clamor with fast-food madness, you don't have to settle for the solitary soggy, cold French fry at the bottom of their take-out bags. You can enjoy the ride—and eat the 5-Day Miracle Diet way, too!

✔ Make it Burger King instead of McDonald's. The operative word is "flame-broiled."

✔ Ask for all the veggie extras you can think of on your "Have It Your Way" burger: Onions, lettuce, and tomato can really fill you up!

✔ Try mustard and pickles instead of "special sauce," which has lots of sugar and fat. And as we all know, no sugar, no cravings.

✔ Stick to unsweetened iced tea or that old-fashioned drink they call "water."

• •

"Everything you see I owe to spaghetti."

—*Sophia Loren*

If only we were all so blessed!

• •

> *"If you eat a protein and a starch every morning, you'll be on the road to good blood sugar. Like the 'good, hot breakfast' of yore, it sticks to you, especially after you've eaten that first hard chew."*
>
> —*The Daily Adele Dose*

● ●

Date:

What I ate...for breakfast: _____

_____

_____

What I ate...for my morning hard-chew snacks: _____

_____

What I ate...for lunch: _____

_____

_____

_____

What I ate...for my afternoon soft chews: _____

What I ate...for dinner:_____

_____

_____

_____

How I felt: _____

_____

_____

How I kept moving: _____

_____

_____

What I drank: _____

_____

*Did I eat a protein and a starch for breakfast?*_____

> *"I not only learned how to eat on the 5-Day Miracle Diet. I learned how to live!"*
>
> —A twenty-year-old college student

MELON MADNESS

The Japanese grow some of the most succulent, delicious melons in the world. Their farming methods might not be the most profitable, but they produce the sweetest fruit.

Japanese farmers plant a seed, allowing it to grow and form buds. They then pick all the buds—except one. This one bud grows into maturity, into full fruit, receiving all the nutrients and all the attention that had originally been produced for all the buds. The result? One fabulous melon that's as expensive and considered as luxurious as the best champagne!

The lesson? Nurture yourself and you, too, can be fabulous!

"Instead of concentrating on the numbers on the scale, think of how your clothes are getting looser and you're looking trimmer!"

—*The Daily Adele Dose*

• •

Date: _____

What I ate...for breakfast: _____
_____
_____

What I ate...for my morning hard-chew snacks: _____
_____

What I ate...for lunch: _____
_____
_____
_____

What I ate...for my afternoon soft chews: _____

What I ate...for dinner: _____
_____
_____
_____

How I felt: _____
_____
_____

How I kept moving: _____
_____
_____

What I drank: _____
_____

Did I alter some clothing so that I don't have that "someone who's just lost a lot of weight and is wearing baggy clothes" look?
_____

GREEN-TOTIN' MEN AND WOMEN

Since vegetables are such a crucial part of the 5-Day Miracle Diet, I've devised ways to make toting those carrots and string beans easy—and keeping them fresh and crunchy, too!

Keep a Post-It on your inside doorway. As you're running out the door, you won't forget to pick up one of your perforated bags of hard chews to take to work.

Another "forget-me-not" I learned from my husband. He puts a Post-It right on the handle of his attaché case the night before.

An excerpt from a letter I received from a thirtysomething man who'd just read my book:

"I couldn't contain my excitement. I had to write to say that you changed my life. Literally! Before I read your book I was an overweight failure. Now I feel like an overweight winner—and I'm doing something about the overweight part, too! Thank you, Adele."

"My diet is the single most powerful thing you can give yourself. It will follow you into every aspect of your life!"

—The Daily Adele Dose

• •

Date:

What I ate...for breakfast: _____
_____
_____

What I ate...for my morning hard-chew snacks: _____
_____

What I ate...for lunch: _____
_____
_____
_____

What I ate...for my afternoon soft chews: _____

What I ate...for dinner: _____
_____
_____
_____

How I felt: _____
_____
_____

How I kept moving: _____
_____
_____

What I drank: _____
_____

Did I feel confident today? _____

A Personal Mantra

I have a confession to make: Sometimes after a day filled with interviews, television shows, and book signings, I'm tired. Even my good blood sugar can't stop the weariness that comes after these long, exciting days.

The weariness really got to me one day when I was on a cross-country book tour. I had just done four back-to-back interviews and I was due to go on a live television show in five minutes. I was so distracted that I was afraid the great enthusiasm I felt for my program and for my clients wouldn't be expressed on the air.

My husband came to the rescue. He put his arm around me and said, "Adele, just relax. Go out there and have fun."

I nodded. I took a deep breath. And then I smiled. He was right! Forget the long hours. Forget the hot lights. Just go out there and have a good time.

So now, whenever I'm about to go out on stage or into a studio for an interview, I simply say to myself, "Have fun." And I do. The smiling face you see on the screen is mine!

The moral? Reward yourself with the same words—and actions. Go out there and have fun!

"Why isn't everyone on the 5-Day Miracle Diet? Who knows? Maybe we'd have the stamina to find world peace!"

—*The Daily Adele Dose*

• •

Date:

What I ate...for breakfast: _____
_____
_____

What I ate...for my morning hard-chew snacks: _____
_____

What I ate...for lunch: _____
_____
_____
_____

What I ate...for my afternoon soft chews: _____

What I ate...for dinner:_____
_____
_____
_____

How I felt: _____
_____
_____

How I kept moving: _____
_____
_____

What I drank: _____
_____

Did I write down the natural exercise I did today? _____

FIT FOR A KING

Louis XIV of France, the famous "Sun King" of Versailles, had a stomach twice the size of a normal man's. It's no wonder. An average dinner for him consisted of four hearty plates of soup, an entire pheasant, one big partridge, two huge slices of ham, mutton cooked with garlic, pastries, fruit, hard-boiled eggs, and, lest he forget his health, a nice salad.

EXERCISE WILL:

- Jump-start your metabolism
- Burn calories even after you've finished
- Keep up a steady weight loss on the 5-Day Miracle Diet
- Help slow down osteoporosis
- Reduce stress
- Tone muscles
- Increase the good cholesterol (HDL), which is vital for strong, healthy hearts
- Make you look and feel great!

"Good blood sugar sounds so easy—and so unconnected to feeling empowered. And yet the connection is so powerful, so immediate, that you will notice it right away."

—*The Daily Adele Dose*

• •

Date: _____

What I ate...for breakfast: _____
_____
_____

What I ate...for my morning hard-chew snacks: _____
_____

What I ate...for lunch: _____
_____
_____
_____

What I ate...for my afternoon soft chews: _____

What I ate...for dinner: _____
_____
_____
_____

How I felt: _____
_____
_____

How I kept moving: _____
_____
_____

What I drank: _____
_____

Did I wake up without that usual anxious, knots-in-the-stomach feeling? _____

WEEKLY ASSESSMENT

WEIGHTY ISSUES

Last week's weight: _____

Pounds lost: _____

New weight: _____

Don't forget those lost ounces and half pounds. They add up!

● ●

Instead of heading for the cookies, head for your appointment book—and schedule a haircut, a massage, a facial, or a tennis game. You'll feel fabulous long after the "need" for the cookie is gone!

● ●

A WEEK'S "POCKETFUL OF MIRACLES"

It's hard to believe that we've traveled together, through thick and thin, for almost six months. I am profoundly moved that so many of you have decided to try to change your lives—and that so many of you have gone out there and done it!

But now, as we stroll toward our goal, it's important to remember that you yourself are the miracle behind my diet plan. The rewards belong to you. *You* made it happen. I was just around to help and understand.

So before you write your last entry in this section, go back to that very first week, and see what you wrote as your goal. Did you make it? Did you surpass it? Or did it change along the way?

It's time now to write a new goal, one that will take you into the future. Here's an entry from one of my clients:

● *Today, I begin my next six months, on my own—and "owning" the diet. My goal is to translate the empowerment I feel with food into my life. Why not? I always wanted to take a watercolor course and run a marathon, too!*

Now it's your turn: _____

_____

_____

"Just think. Every time you pass up a fattening dessert or main dish because you don't want it, it's a miracle—that you made happen. You! The person who didn't have any control when it came to 'craving the crave'!"

—*The Daily Adele Dose*

• •

Date:

What I ate...for breakfast:_____

_____

What I ate...for my morning hard-chew snacks:_____

_____

What I ate...for lunch:_____

_____

_____

What I ate...for my afternoon soft chews:_____

What I ate...for dinner:_____

_____

_____

How I felt:_____

_____

How I kept moving:_____

_____

What I drank:_____

Did I try jazzing up my salad with exotic greens and other veggies?

_____

THE DEVIL MADE ME DO IT

This is one of my favorite stories—and one I tell my new clients over and over again. It's about Danny, a tall, strapping man with a joie de vivre about him. He was bigger than life; he loved his family, his work, his leisure time, and, of course, his food. He did everything passionately—and excessively.

By the time he was in his forties, he was forty pounds overweight.

When I explained how simple the 5-Day Miracle Diet was, he couldn't believe me at first, but he agreed to try. Everything went great for the first two weeks. Then things changed. Danny started gaining weight. He struggled all the time.

But he wasn't unhappy about the situation—an unusual reaction, to say the least. In fact, he was just as passionate and lively as ever. He came bounding into my office ready to describe in tantalizing detail the fabulous steak he had had the night before, grilled to perfection. He couldn't wait to tell me about the pasta dish at the new restaurant near his apartment—one made with heavy cream, of course! Then there were the desserts, each more scrumptious than the one before.

I asked Danny point-blank, "Why? Why aren't you following the program?"

Danny always said the same thing, with a big, fat grin on his face: "The devil made me do it."

Although he was kidding, Danny wasn't far off the mark. There really is a "devil" that makes us eat. As all of you know by now, it's called low blood sugar—and its only cure is the 5-Day Miracle Diet.

"Losing weight has nothing to do with deprivation!"
—*The Daily Adele Dose*

• •

Date:

What I ate...for breakfast: _____
_____
_____

What I ate...for my morning hard-chew snacks: _____
_____

What I ate...for lunch: _____
_____
_____
_____

What I ate...for my afternoon soft chews: _____

What I ate...for dinner: _____
_____
_____
_____

How I felt: _____
_____
_____

How I kept moving: _____
_____
_____

What I drank: _____
_____

Did I successfully handle a fathead *issue?* _____

"THE DEVIL MADE ME DO IT" CHOCOLATE CAKE
THE SPECIALTY OF RESTAURANT NAVONA

Close your eyes. Imagine the most sinfully delicious, indescribably sweet, melt-in-your-mouth chocolate fantasy and you might get close—just close—to this incredible dessert. Named after "The Devil Made Me Do It" Danny, my bigger-than-life client who would appreciate this heavenly concoction to the max, I offer it here as the "Ultimate Extra." It's a treat you will absolutely adore. But remember my Four Rules of Selectivity!

And eater beware: You will feel the effects of this dessert well after you've put down your fork; your sugar cravings will be in full force and you'll need two days of steady GBS to calm yourself down.

On the other hand, life is for loving, living, and enjoying every single, solitary bite—and that includes this luscious chocolate cake. So for a super-special "Extra"... enjoy. To life!

What you'll need:

1½ pounds semisweet chocolate bits or squares
 ½ cup (1 stick) unsalted butter, at room temperature
 6 eggs, separated
 6 tablespoons sugar
 3 tablespoons flour
    Whipped cream, for serving (optional)

What you'll do:

Preheat the oven to 400°F.

Melt the chocolate in a double boiler. When the chocolate is thoroughly melted, add the butter. Melt the butter in the chocolate. Remove from the heat.

Add the egg yolks, sugar, and flour and mix thoroughly using a hand beater.

Beat the egg whites separately until foamy. Gently fold the egg whites into the chocolate mixture.

Pour the batter into a 12-inch springform pan and bake for 25 minutes. Remove sides of pan and slice. Serve warm with whipped cream, if desired.

Serves anywhere from 1 to 12. I hope you'll be with a chocolate-hungry crowd!

"I've done all the work for you on the diet. All you have to do is give me a five-day commitment and the rest will be easy!"

—*The Daily Adele Dose*

• •

Date:

What I ate...for breakfast: _____

_____

_____

What I ate...for my morning hard-chew snacks: _____

_____

What I ate...for lunch: _____

_____

_____

_____

What I ate...for my afternoon soft chews: _____

What I ate...for dinner: _____

_____

_____

_____

How I felt: _____

_____

_____

How I kept moving: _____

_____

_____

What I drank: _____

_____

Did I try eating crudités with one of my dip recipes for a change-of-pace snack? _____

NEVER SAY GOODBYE

The 5-Day Miracle Diet is not about never eating certain things ever again. It's not about saying goodbye to breads and cheeses and chocolate soufflé. What the 5-Day Miracle Diet is all about is learning how to live with your foods, not without them!

TAKE ME OUT TO THE BALL GAME

That three-base hit is definitely cause for celebration (if it's your team!), but cheers don't have to be shouted over drafts of beer. While sitting in the bleachers might work up an appetite, there are other treats besides hot dogs smothered in fried onions, cotton candy, and beer. How about popcorn—sans the butter? Or a hot dog with mustard and sauerkraut? (You can even use the roll as a "napkin," eating just the dog and cutting back on the calories!) And how about a cold iced tea or that clear liquid they call water?

Remember, if you're really into your team, you're having a ball, and most important, you're in good blood sugar, go for that sip of cold beer. You earned it—once or twice a week.

"Isn't it a great feeling to have control over your own life? That's what the 5-Day Miracle Diet gives you!"

—*The Daily Adele Dose*

• •

Date:

What I ate...for breakfast: _____
_____
_____

What I ate...for my morning hard-chew snacks: _____
_____

What I ate...for lunch: _____
_____
_____
_____

What I ate...for my afternoon soft chews: _____

What I ate...for dinner: _____
_____
_____
_____

How I felt: _____
_____
_____

How I kept moving: _____
_____
_____

What I drank: _____
_____

Did I try an exotic vinegar on my salad instead of dressing?
_____

"When you're hungry, sing. When you're hurt, laugh."

—*Jewish proverb*

TRUE PHYSICAL HUNGER VS.
"FEED ME" *FATHEAD* CRAVINGS

True physical hunger occurs three to four hours after your last meal or snack.

Cravings come on at any time, day or night.

True physical hunger lasts for twenty minutes, during which time the stomach contracts and the body begins to use stored energy.

Cravings can pass in seconds—or last for "white-knuckled" days on end.

True physical hunger is an automatic physiological response.

Cravings can be both a physiological response to blood-sugar imbalance—or triggered by emotional cues.

"My 5-Day Miracle Diet didn't happen by accident. I spent years perfecting it so that I could enthusiastically and happily share it with you!"

—*The Daily Adele Dose*

• •

Date:

What I ate...for breakfast: _____

_____

_____

What I ate...for my morning hard-chew snacks: _____

_____

What I ate...for lunch: _____

_____

_____

_____

What I ate...for my afternoon soft chews: _____

What I ate...for dinner: _____

_____

_____

_____

How I felt: _____

_____

_____

How I kept moving: _____

_____

_____

What I drank: _____

_____

*Did I do a few stomach crunches or some push-ups today?*_____

IDLE MINDS, IDLE HANDS

One of the best ways to keep from eating is to keep your hands busy. It's difficult to pick up that fork (or that bagel) if your hands—and mind—are elsewhere.

Here are some noncaloric goodies to keep you busy:

- *Kissing*
- Playing the piano
- Knitting
- Putting on fingernail polish
- Washing the car
- Shooting some hoops
- Gardening
- Driving to the park
- Playing a computer game
- *And, of course,* **Kissing!**

"Seeing you change. That is the greatest gift you can give me!"

—*The Daily Adele Dose*

● ●

Date:

What I ate...for breakfast: _____

_____

What I ate...for my morning hard-chew snacks: _____

_____

What I ate...for lunch: _____

_____

_____

_____

What I ate...for my afternoon soft chews: _____

What I ate...for dinner: _____

_____

_____

_____

How I felt: _____

_____

_____

How I kept moving: _____

_____

_____

What I drank: _____

_____

Did I wake up feeling refreshed and in control of my life? _____

A SHARED MOMENT:
IT'S THE PEOPLE WHO COUNT

At an early book signing, I was going to start speaking about the simplicity and ease of the 5-Day Miracle Diet when I stopped short. Suddenly, I noticed the faces around me—of men, women, teens, young adults, and those my age and older. These faces, over one hundred in all, were looking up at me from their chairs and from their seats cross-legged on the floor.

They were looking at me with hope in their eyes. They were expectant and excited.

And that's when I profoundly understood what this was all about—the tours, the talks, the interviews, and the shows: It was all about the people, the connection between them and me and you, and how, with a simple diet plan, I could help people change their own lives dramatically.

This was the miracle.

I began to speak with a new surge of profound gratitude and energy.

Thank you all!

"I can help you keep your excess weight off forever. "
                                                    —*The Daily Adele Dose*

• •

Date:

What I ate...for breakfast: _____

_____

_____

What I ate...for my morning hard-chew snacks: _____

_____

What I ate...for lunch: _____

_____

_____

_____

What I ate...for my afternoon soft chews: _____

What I ate...for dinner: _____

_____

_____

_____

How I felt: _____

_____

_____

How I kept moving: _____

_____

_____

What I drank: _____

_____

Did I follow my basic diet plan today? _____

SIX MONTHS OF MIRACLES

*O*nce again, congratulations are in order. You've finished six full months on the 5-Day Miracle Diet. Before we close, although it's not necessary, here's a last time to record inches and weight:

Inch-by-Inch

Bust/chest: _____   Upper arms: _____

Wrists: _____   Waist: _____

Abdomen: _____   Hips and buttocks: _____

WEIGHTY ISSUES

Last week's weight: _____

Pounds lost: _____

New Weight: _____

Don't forget those lost ounces and half pounds. They add up!

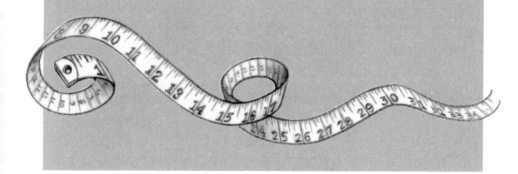

Keep soaring, keep going.
Keep reaching for your goals.
To all the miracles in your life
that await you!

SOURCES

Almada, Anthony. "Sweet Talk and Bittersweet Truths." *Natural Healing*, March 1992.

Brownell, Kelly D., Ph.D. *The Learn Program for Weight Control*, Sixth Edition. Dallas, Texas: American Health Publishing Company, 1994.

Hirsch, Cheryl. "Blood Sugar and Brain Function." *Medical Nutrition*, Summer 1989.

Nowlan, Mary Hegarty, and Elizabeth Hiser. "The Hungry Mind." *Eating Well*, May–June 1995.

Puhn, Adele. *The 5-Day Miracle Diet*. New York: Ballantine Books, Inc., 1996.

Rippe, Dr. James M., and Ann Ward, Ph.D., with Karla Dougherty. *The Rockport Walking Program*. New York: Fireside, 1989.

Russo, Julee, and Sheila Lukins. *The New Basics*. New York: Workman Publishing, 1989.

Shapiro, Laura. "Food Lover's Guide to Fat." *Newsweek*, December 5, 1994.

Ulene, Dr. Art. *The Nutribase Guide to Carbohydrates, Calories, & Fat in Your Food*. Garden City, New York: Avery Publishing Group, 1995.

_____. *The Nutribase Guide to Fat & Cholesterol in Your Food*. Garden City, New York: Avery Publishing Group, 1995.

Waterhouse, Debra, M.P.H., R.D. *Why Women Need Chocolate*. New York: Hyperion, 1995.

ABOUT THE AUTHOR

ADELE PUHN, M.S., C.N.S., has been a nutritional consultant for eighteen years with a thriving private practice both on the Upper East Side of New York and in Great Neck, Long Island. Her patients run the gamut from the rich and famous (who will not be mentioned here) to more ordinary folk.

She holds an M.S. in Medical Biology and a Certificate in Clinical Nutrition and is a Certified Nutrition Specialist as conferred by the American College of Nutrition. Recently appointed the nutritional advisor of Self-Help, an agency that helps the families of mothers with AIDS stay together, she is also a frequent lecturer at seminars and conferences, and has worked at various health centers and with school systems on Long Island. Her nutrition and weight-loss research has made her a popu-lar source for magazines, and her thoughts and ideas have appeared in *Mirabella*, *Harper's Bazaar*, and *The Wall Street Journal*. She is the author of the *New York Times* bestseller, *The 5-Day Miracle Diet*.

Ms. Puhn lives in the Kensington section of Great Neck, Long Island, with her husband. Her grown children frequently visit—and none of them crave Twinkies when they do.